Curing Diabetes Naturally

Table of Contents

Chapter 1

Types of diabetes

You can figure out how to deal with your diabetes and keep a percentage of the significant issues diabetes can bring about. The more you know, the better you can deal with your diabetes. Offer this booklet with your family and companions so they will see more about diabetes. Likewise try to ask your social insurance group any inquiries you may have.

You can figure out how to deal with your diabetes.

Diabetes is the point at which your blood glucose, additionally called glucose, is too high. Blood glucose is the principle type of sugar found in your blood and your fundamental wellspring of vitality. Glucose originates from the nourishment you eat and is additionally made in your liver and muscles. Your blood conveys glucose to the greater part of your body's cells to use for vitality.

Your pancreas—an organ, situated between your stomach and spine, that assists with processing—discharges a hormone it makes, called insulin, into your blood. Insulin offers your blood some assistance with carrying glucose to all your body's cells. Here and there your body doesn't make enough insulin or the insulin doesn't work the way it ought to. Glucose then stays in your blood and doesn't achieve your cells. Your blood glucose levels get too high and can bring about diabetes or prediabetes.

After some time, having an excess of glucose in your blood can bring about wellbeing issues.

Prediabetes is the point at which the measure of glucose in your blood is above typical yet not sufficiently high to be called diabetes. With prediabetes, your odds of getting type 2 diabetes, coronary illness, and stroke are higher. With some weight reduction and moderate physical action, you can defer or anticipate type 2 diabetes. You can even come back to typical glucose levels, conceivably without taking any prescriptions. Drawing of a stoplight with the words Caution: Take ventures to counteract type 2 diabetes now.

being exceptionally parched

urinating frequently

feeling exceptionally hungry

feeling exceptionally drained

shedding pounds without attempting

wounds that recuperate gradually

dry, bothersome skin

sentiments of pins and needles in your feet

losing feeling in your feet

hazy visual perception

A few individuals with diabetes don't have any of these signs or side effects. The best way to know whether you have diabetes is to have your specialist do a blood test.

What type of diabetes do you have?

The three principle types of diabetes are type 1, type 2, and gestational diabetes. Individuals can create diabetes at any age. Both ladies and men can create diabetes.

Type 1 Diabetes

Type 1 diabetes, which used to be called adolescent diabetes, grows regularly in youngsters; be that as it may, type 1 diabetes can likewise create in grown-ups. In type 1 diabetes, your body no more makes insulin or enough insulin on the grounds that the body's resistant framework, which typically shields you from disease by disposing of microbes, infections, and other destructive substances, has assaulted and crushed the phones that make insulin.

Treatment for type 1 diabetes incorporates

taking shots, additionally called infusions, of insulin.

in some cases taking prescriptions by mouth.

settling on sound sustenance decisions.

being physically dynamic.

controlling your pulse levels. Circulatory strain is the power of blood stream inside your veins.

controlling your cholesterol levels. Cholesterol is a type of fat in your body's cells, in your blood, and in numerous nourishments.

Type 2 Diabetes

Type 2 diabetes, which used to be called grown-up onset diabetes, can influence individuals at any age, even kids. On the other hand, type 2 diabetes grows frequently in moderately aged and more seasoned individuals. Individuals who are overweight and inert are additionally more prone to create type 2 diabetes.

Type 2 diabetes as a rule starts with insulin resistance—a condition that happens when fat, muscle, and liver cells don't utilize insulin to convey glucose into the body's cells to use for vitality. Thus, the body needs more insulin to offer glucose some assistance with entering cells. At to begin with, the pancreas stays aware of the included interest by making more insulin. Over the long run, the pancreas doesn't make enough insulin when glucose levels expansion, for example, after dinners. If that your pancreas can no more make enough insulin, you should treat your type 2 diabetes.

Treatment for type 2 diabetes incorporates

utilizing diabetes drugs

settling on sound nourishment decisions

being physically dynamic

controlling your pulse levels

controlling your cholesterol levels

Gestational Diabetes

Gestational diabetes can create when a lady is pregnant. Pregnant ladies make hormones that can prompt insulin resistance. All ladies have insulin resistance late in their pregnancy. If that the pancreas doesn't make enough insulin duringpregnancy, a lady creates gestational diabetes. Overweight or stout ladies have a higher possibility of gestational diabetes. Additionally, putting on an excessive amount of weight duringpregnancy might improve your probability of creating gestational diabetes.

Gestational diabetes frequently leaves after the child is conceived. Be that as it may, a lady who has had gestational diabetes will probably create type 2 diabetes further down the road. Babies destined to moms who had gestational diabetes are likewise more inclined to create weight and type 2 diabetes.

More data about diabetes and pregnancy is given in the NIDDK wellbeing theme, What I have to think about Gestational Diabetes.

Why do you have to deal with your diabetes?

After some time, diabetes can prompt difficult issues with your veins, heart, nerves, kidneys, mouth, eyes, and feet. These issues can prompt a removal, which is surgery to uproot a harmed toe, foot, or leg, for instance. The most major issue brought on by diabetes is coronary illness. When you have diabetes, you are more than twice as likely as individuals without diabetes to have coronary illness or a stroke. With diabetes, you might not have the typical signs or indications of a heart assault. The most ideal approach to deal with your wellbeing is to work with your medicinal services group to keep your blood glucose, circulatory strain, and cholesterol levels in your objective extent. Targets are numbers you go for.

Who is a piece of your social insurance group?

A great many people with diabetes get care from essential consideration suppliers, for example, internists, family doctors, or pediatricians. A group of medicinal services suppliers can likewise enhance your diabetes care.

Notwithstanding an essential consideration supplier, your medicinal services group might incorporate

an endocrinologist for more particular diabetes care

a dietitian, a medical caretaker, or an ensured diabetes teacher—specialists who can give data about overseeing diabetes

an instructor or psychological well-being proficient

a drug specialist

a dental specialist

an ophthalmologist or an optometrist for eye care

a podiatrist for foot care

If that diabetes makes you feel miserable or furious, or if that you have different issues that stress you, you ought to converse with an instructor or emotional well-being proficient. Your specialist or ensured diabetes teacher can offer you some assistance with finding a guide.

Converse with your specialist about what antibodies and vaccinations, or shots, you ought to get the chance to keep from becoming ill. Forestalling ailment is an imperative piece of dealing with your diabetes. When you see individuals from your medicinal services group, solicit parts from inquiries. Set up a rundown of inquiries before your visit. Make certain you comprehend all that you have to think about dealing with your diabetes.

Types of Diabetes

In spite of the fact that there are three primary types of diabetes, there is additionally a stage before diabetes called pre-diabetes. Pre-diabetes, otherwise called Impaired glucose resistance is a condition where your Blood sugar level lifts to a level higher than the ordinary reach for a great many people, yet is still sufficiently low not to be considered diabetes. Individuals who have pre-diabetes are at danger of creating Type 2 diabetes further down the road if that they don't screen their condition painstakingly.

Individuals who have been determined to have pre-diabetes can keep from advancing to an out and out watching so as to find of Type 2 diabetes their weight, practicing and eating the right nourishments.

The primary principle type of diabetes is Type 1 diabetes, an Autoimmune infection where the pancreas delivers almost no insulin or no insulin by any stretch of the imagination. Individuals who get Type 1 diabetes are generally less than 20 years old, ordinarily introducing itself when the individual is a tyke or youthful grown-up.

A few researchers trust that Type 1 diabetes is a hereditary condition where the cells of the Pancreas are assaulted and after that quit working. Others feel the illness might be brought about by an infection that provoke the insusceptible framework to start assaulting the pancreas.

Since the pancreas cells that create Insulin are devastated, individuals who create Type 1 diabetes will have the infection forever and will require treatment as insulin shots or an insulin pump. Notwithstanding insulin treatment, exercise and cautious regard for eating routine is important to forestall changes of glucose.

Type 2 diabetes is typically found in individuals who are overweight as they get more established. In spite of the fact that it is now and then called grown-up onset diabetes, in some nation, for example, the United States, more kids and youthful grown-ups are being determined to have Type 2 diabetes since they are not getting enough movement.

Around 90 percent of all instances of diabetes are Type 2 diabetes. The distinction between Type 1 and Type 2 diabetes is that with Type 2 diabetes the pancreas does not sufficiently deliver insulin or the body does not legitimately utilize the it.

Type 2 diabetes is now and then considered a way of life illness since it is regularly activated by carrying on with a genuinely stationary life, being overweight and not partaking in activity. Be that as it may, age is an element and additionally heredity. If that a guardian or kin creates Type 2 diabetes further down the road, a man has more prominent opportunities to getting Type 2 diabetes also.

The third principle type of diabetes is gestational diabetes, which is a condition that ladies can get when they are in the second trimester of pregnancy. Around 4 percent of every pregnant wome will create gestational diabetes. Not at all like Type 1 and Type 2 diabetes, gestational diabetes will vanish after the child is conceived.

At the point when a lady has an event of gestational diabetes duringpregnancy, she will probably have it again in the following pregnancy and puts the lady at a higher danger of creating Type 2 diabetes sometime down the road. The more established a lady is the point at which she is pregnant, the higher the danger of creating gestational diabetes duringpregnancy.

Diabetes is a ceaseless, regularly crippling and some of the time lethal ailment, in which the body either can't deliver insulin or can't appropriately utilize the insulin it produces. Insulin is a hormone that controls the measure of glucose (sugar) in the blood. Diabetes prompts high glucose levels, which can harm organs, veins and nerves. The body needs insulin to utilize sugar as a vitality source.

What is the pancreas ?

The pancreas is an organ that sits behind the stomach and discharges hormones into the digestive framework. In the sound body, when glucose levels get too high, uncommon cells in the pancreas (called beta cells) discharge insulin. Insulin is a hormone and it causes cells to take in sugar to use as vitality or to store as fat. This reasons glucose levels to do a reversal down.

What is type 1 diabetes?

Type 1 diabetes happens when the resistant framework erroneously assaults and slaughters the beta cells of the pancreas. No, or practically nothing, insulin is discharged into the body. Thus, sugar develops in the blood as opposed to being utilized as vitality. Around five to 10 for each penny of individuals with diabetes have type 1 diabetes. Type 1 diabetes by and large creates in youth or pre-adulthood, however can create in adulthood. Type 1 diabetes is constantly treated with insulin. Feast arranging additionally assists with keeping glucose at the right levels. Type 1 diabetes likewise incorporates dormant immune system diabetes in grown-ups (LADA), the term used to portray the little number of individuals with obvious type 2 diabetes who seem to have insusceptible intervened loss of pancreatic beta cells.

What is type 2 diabetes?

Type 2 diabetes happens when the body can't legitimately utilize the insulin that is discharged (called insulin lack of care) or does not make enough insulin. Thus, sugar develops in the blood as opposed to being utilized as vitality. Around 90 for each penny of individuals with diabetes have type 2 diabetes. Type 2 diabetes all the more frequently creates in grown-ups, however youngsters can be influenced.

Contingent upon the seriousness of type 2 diabetes, it might be overseen through physical action and dinner arranging, or might likewise require medicines and/or insulin to control glucose all the more viably.

What is gestational diabetes?

A third type of diabetes, gestational diabetes, is an interim condition that happens during pregnancy. It influences roughly two to four for each penny of all pregnancies (in the non-Aboriginal populace) and includes an greater danger of creating diabetes for both mother and tyke.

What are the problems associated with diabetes?

Having high glucose can bring about diabetes-related intricacies, as endless kidney sickness, foot issues, non-traumatic lower appendage (leg, foot, toe, and so on.) removal, eye malady (retinopathy) that can prompt visual impairment, heart assault, stroke, uneasiness, nerve harm, and erectile brokenness (men).

Diabetes-related entanglements can be intense and even life-undermining. Legitimately overseeing glucose levels lessens the danger of adding to these complexities.

Chapter 2

Symptoms of diabetes

Early indications of diabetes, particularly type 2 diabetes, can be unobtrusive or apparently safe — if that you have side effects by any means. After some time, be that as it may, you might create diabetes difficulties, regardless of the possibility that you haven't had diabetes side effects.

In the United States alone, almost 7 million individuals have undiscovered diabetes, as indicated by the American Diabetes Association. Be that as it may, you don't have to end up a measurement. Understanding conceivable diabetes indications can prompt early analysis and treatment — and a lifetime of better wellbeing. In case you're encountering any of the accompanying diabetes signs and side effects, see your specialist.

Extreme thirst and frequent urination

Extreme thirst and greater pee are great diabetes side effects.

When you have diabetes, abundance sugar (glucose) develops in your blood. Your kidneys are compelled to work additional time to channel and ingest the overabundance sugar. If that your kidneys can't keep up, the abundance sugar is discharged into your pee alongside liquids drawn from your tissues. This triggers more successive pee, which might abandon you got dried out. As you drink more liquids to extinguish your thirst, you'll urinate much more

Weakness

You might feel exhausted. Numerous elements can add to this. They incorporate parchedness from greater pee and your body's failure to work legitimately, since it's less ready to utilize sugar for vitality needs.

Weight reduction

Weight vacillations likewise fall under the umbrella of conceivable diabetes signs and manifestations. When you lose sugar through successive pee, you likewise lose calories. In the meantime, diabetes might keep the sugar from your sustenance from coming to your cells — prompting consistent appetite. The consolidated impact is possibly quick weight reduction, particularly if that you have type 1 diabetes.

Loss of vision

Diabetes indications here and there include your vision. Abnormal amounts of glucose force liquid from your tissues, including the lenses of your eyes. This influences your capacity to center. Left untreated, diabetes can cause fresh recruits vessels to shape in your retina — the back a portion of your eye — and harm set up vessels. For a great many people, these early changes don't cause vision issues. On the other hand, if these progressions progress undetected, they can prompt vision misfortune and visual impairment.

Specialists and individuals with diabetes have watched that contaminations appear to be more regular if that you have diabetes. Research here, then again, has not demonstrated whether this is completely genuine, nor why. It might be that abnormal amounts of glucose debilitate your body's normal mending process and your capacity to battle diseases. For ladies, bladder and vaginal contaminations are particularly regular.

Trembling hands and feet

Abundance sugar in your blood can prompt nerve harm. You might see shivering and loss of sensation in your grasp and feet, and also blazing torment in your arms, hands, legs and feet.

Red, swollen, delicate gums

Diabetes might debilitate your capacity to battle germs, which builds the danger of disease in your gums and in the bones that hold your teeth set up. Your gums might pull far from your teeth, your teeth might turn out to be free, or you might create injuries or pockets of discharge in your gums — particularly if that you have a gum contamination before diabetes develops.

Consider your body's clues important

If that you see any conceivable diabetes signs or indications, contact your specialist. The prior the condition is analyzed, the sooner treatment can start. Diabetes is a genuine condition. In any case, with your dynamic investment and the backing of your human services group, you can oversee diabetes while appreciating a dynamic approach. By what means would you be able to tell if that you have diabetes? Most early indications are from higher-than-typical levels of glucose, a sort of sugar, in your blood.

The notice signs can be mild to the point that you don't see them. That is particularly valid for type 2 diabetes. A few individuals don't discover they have it until they get issues from long haul harm caused by the malady. With type 1 diabetes, the indications for the most part happen rapidly, in a matter of days or a couple of weeks. They're substantially more extreme, as well.

Hunger and weakness. Your body changes over the nourishment you eat into glucose that your cells use for vitality. In any case, your phones need insulin to acquire the glucose. If that your body doesn't make enough or any insulin, or if your cells oppose the insulin your body makes, the glucose can't get into them and you have no vitality. This can make you more eager and tired than expected.

Peeing all the more regularly and being thirstier. The normal individual more often than not needs to pee somewhere around four and seven times in 24 hours, however individuals with diabetes might go significantly more. Why? Regularly your body reabsorbs glucose as it goes through your kidneys. In any case, when diabetes pushes your glucose up, your body will be unable to get it all back. It will attempt to dispose of the additional by making more pee, and that takes liquids.

You'll need to go all the more regularly. You may pee out all the more, as well. Because you're peeing so much, you can get extremely parched. When you drink more, you'll likewise pee more. Dry mouth and bothersome skin. Because your body is utilizing liquids to make pee, there's less dampness for different things. You could get got dried out, and your mouth might feel dry. Dry skin can make you irritated.

 Changing liquid levels in your body could make the lenses in your eyes swell up. They change shape and lose their capacity to center.

Other Type 2 Symptoms

These tend to appear after your glucose has been high for quite a while.

Yeast diseases. Both men and ladies with diabetes can get these. Yeast sustains on glucose, so having bounty around makes it flourish.

Contaminations can develop in any warm, sodden fold of skin, including:

In the middle of fingers and toes

Under arms

In or around sex organs

Moderate mending injuries or cuts. After some time, high glucose can influence your blood stream and cause nerve harm that makes it hard for your body to mend wounds. Torment or deadness in your feet or legs. This is another aftereffect of nerve harm. related substance

Spontaneous weight reduction. If that your body can't get vitality from your nourishment, it will begin blazing muscle and fat for vitality. You might get more fit despite the fact that you haven't changed how you eat. Queasiness and regurgitating. At the point when your body resorts to blazing fat, it makes "ketones." These can develop in your blood to unsafe levels, a potentially life-undermining condition called diabetic ketoacidosis. Ketones can make you feel wiped out to your stomach.

In case you're more seasoned than 45 or have different dangers for diabetes, it's essential to get tried. When you recognize the condition early, you can maintain a strategic distance from nerve harm, heart inconvenience, and different entanglements.

When in doubt, call your specialist if that you:

Feel wiped out to your stomach, powerless, and extremely parched

Are peeing a great deal

Have an awful complain

Are breathing more profoundly and speedier than ordinary

Have sweet breath that possesses an aroma similar to nail shine remover. (This is an indication of high ketones.

Chapter 3

What causes type 1 diabetes?

Type 1 diabetes is caused by an absence of insulin because of the devastation of insulin-creating beta cells in the pancreas. In type 1 diabetes—an immune system ailment—the body's safe framework assaults and wrecks the beta cells. Ordinarily, the invulnerable framework shields the body from contamination by recognizing and obliterating microscopic organisms, infections, and other possibly destructive outside substances. In any case, in immune system ailments, the invulnerable framework assaults the body's own cells. In type 1 diabetes, beta cell devastation might happen more than quite a while, yet indications of the infection as a rule create over a brief timeframe.

Type 1 diabetes ordinarily happens in youngsters and youthful grown-ups, however it can show up at any age. Previously, type 1 diabetes was called adolescent diabetes or insulin-subordinate diabetes mellitus.

Inactive immune system diabetes in grown-ups (LADA) might be a gradually creating sort of type 1 diabetes. Analysis more often than not happens after age 30. In LADA, as in type 1 diabetes, the body's resistant framework wrecks the beta cells. At the season of analysis, individuals with LADA might in any case create their own particular insulin, yet in the end most will need insulin shots or an insulin pump to control blood glucose levels.

Genetic vulnerability

Heredity has critical impact in figuring out why should likely create type 1 diabetes. Qualities are gone down from natural guardian to youngster. Qualities convey directions for making proteins that are required for the body's cells to work. Numerous qualities, and in addition communications among qualities, are thought to impact weakness to and insurance from type 1 diabetes. The key qualities might fluctuate in various populace bunches. Varieties in qualities that influence more than 1 percent of a populace gathering are called quality variations.

Certain quality variations that convey guidelines for making proteins called human leukocyte antigens (HLAs) on white platelets are connected to the danger of creating type 1 diabetes. The proteins created by HLA qualities figure out if the insusceptible framework perceives a cell as a component of the body or as remote material. A few mixes of HLA quality variations foresee that a man will be at higher danger for type 1 diabetes, while different mixes are defensive or have no impact on danger.

While HLA qualities are the real hazard qualities for type 1 diabetes, numerous extra hazard qualities or quality locales have been found. Not just can these qualities distinguish individuals at danger for type 1 diabetes, yet they likewise give imperative insights to offer researchers better some assistance with understanding how the malady creates and recognize potential focuses for treatment and counteractive action. Hereditary testing can demonstrate what types of HLA qualities a man conveys and can uncover different qualities connected to diabetes. Then again, most hereditary testing is done in an exploration setting and is not yet accessible to people. Researchers are concentrate how the consequences of hereditary testing can be utilized to enhance type 1 diabetes avoidance or treatment.

Immune system Destruction of Beta Cells

In type 1 diabetes, white platelets called T cells assault and devastate beta cells. The procedure starts well before diabetes side effects show up and proceeds after conclusion. Frequently, type 1 diabetes is not analyzed until most beta cells have as of now been pulverized. As of right now, a man needs day by day insulin treatment to survive. Discovering approaches to change or stop this immune system prepare and save beta cell capacity is a noteworthy center of ebb and flow investigative examination.

Late research recommends insulin itself might be a key trigger of the resistant assault on beta cells. The safe frameworks of individuals why should helpless creating type 1 diabetes react to insulin as though it were a remote substance, or antigen. To battle antigens, the body makes proteins called antibodies. Antibodies to insulin and different proteins created by beta cells are found in individuals with type 1 diabetes. Scientists test for these antibodies to recognize individuals at greater danger of building up the sickness. Testing the types and levels of antibodies in the blood can figure out if a man has type 1 diabetes, LADA, or another type of diabetes.

Environmental factors

Ecological elements, for example, sustenances, infections, and poisons, might assume a part in the advancement of type 1 diabetes, yet the accurate way of their part has not been resolved. A few speculations recommend that natural variables trigger the immune system devastation of beta cells in individuals with a hereditary powerlessness to diabetes. Different hypotheses recommend that natural components assume a continuous part in diabetes, even after determination.

Infections and contaminations. An infection can't cause diabetes all alone, however individuals are once in a while determined to have type 1 diabetes during or after a viral contamination, recommending a connection between the two. Additionally, the onset of type 1 diabetes happens all the more every now and again during the winter when viral contaminations are more regular. Infections perhaps connected with type 1 diabetes incorporate coxsackievirus B, cytomegalovirus, adenovirus, rubella, and mumps. Researchers have depicted a few ways these infections might harm or crush beta cells or conceivably trigger an immune system reaction in defenseless individuals. For instance, hostile to islet antibodies have been found in patients with inborn rubella disorder, and cytomegalovirus has been connected with noteworthy beta cell harm and intense pancreatitis—inflammation of the pancreas. Researchers are attempting to recognize an infection that can cause type 1 diabetes so that an antibody may be created to keep the sickness.

Newborn child bolstering hones. A few studies have recommended that dietary elements might raise or bring down the danger of creating type 1 diabetes. For instance, breastfed babies and newborn children getting vitamin D supplements might have a lessened danger of creating type 1 diabetes, while early introduction to dairy animals' milk and oat proteins might increment hazard. More research is expected to illuminate how newborn child nourishment influences the danger for type 1 diabetes. Perused more in the Centers for Disease Control and Prevention's (CDC's) distribution National Diabetes Statistics Report, 2014 at www.cdc.govExternal Link Disclaimer for data about examination concentrates on identified with type 1 diabetes. What causes type 2 diabetes?

Type 2 diabetes—the most widely recognized type of diabetes—is caused by a blend of variables, including insulin resistance, a condition in which the body's muscle, fat, and liver cells don't utilize insulin viably. Type 2 diabetes creates when the body can no more sufficiently deliver insulin to make up for the debilitated capacity to utilize insulin. Side effects of type 2 diabetes might grow continuously and can be unobtrusive; a few individuals with type 2 diabetes stay undiscovered for a considerable length of time.

Type 2 diabetes grows frequently in moderately aged and more established individuals who are additionally overweight or fat. The ailment, once uncommon in youth, is turning out to be more normal in overweight and stout kids and young people. Researchers think hereditary defenselessness and natural components are the probably triggers of type 2 diabetes. Qualities have noteworthy impact in helplessness to type 2 diabetes. Having certain qualities or mixes of qualities might increment or diminish a man's danger for adding to the infection. The part of qualities is recommended by the high rate of type 2 diabetes in families and indistinguishable twins and wide varieties in diabetes pervasiveness by ethnicity. Type 2 diabetes happens all the more every now and again in African Americans, Alaska Natives, American Indians, Hispanics/Latinos, and some Asian Americans, Native Hawaiians, and Pacific Islander Americans than it does in non-Hispanic whites.

Late studies have joined hereditary information from vast quantities of individuals, quickening the pace of quality disclosure. In spite of the fact that researchers have now recognized numerous quality variations that build defenselessness to type 2 diabetes, the lion's share have yet to be found. The known qualities seem to influence insulin generation as opposed to insulin resistance. Specialists are attempting to recognize extra quality variations and to figure out how they interface with each other and with natural elements to cause diabetes.

Concentrates on have demonstrated that variations of the TCF7L2 quality expand vulnerability to type 2 diabetes. For individuals who acquire two duplicates of the variations, the danger of creating type 2 diabetes is around 80 percent higher than for the individuals who don't convey the quality variant.1 However, even in those with the variation, diet and physical movement prompting weight reduction delay diabetes, as indicated by the Diabetes Prevention Program (DPP), a noteworthy clinical trial including individuals at high hazard.

Qualities can likewise expand the danger of diabetes by expanding a man's propensity to end up overweight or stout. One hypothesis, known as the "thrifty quality" theory, proposes certain qualities expand the proficiency of digestion system to concentrate vitality from nourishment and store the vitality for later utilize. This survival characteristic was profitable for populaces whose nourishment supplies were rare or erratic and could keep individuals alive during starvation. In cutting edge times, on the other hand, when fatty nourishments are abundant, such a quality can advance stoutness and type 2 diabetes.

Heftiness and Physical Inactivity
Physical idleness and corpulence are unequivocally connected with the improvement of type 2 diabetes. Individuals who are hereditarily defenseless to type 2 diabetes are more powerless when these danger

components are available. A lopsidedness between caloric admission and physical action can prompt weight, which causes insulin resistance and is regular in individuals with type 2 diabetes. Focal weight, in which a man has abundance stomach fat, is a noteworthy danger component not just for insulin resistance and type 2 diabetes additionally for heart and vein sickness, likewise called cardiovascular ailment (CVD). This overabundance "stomach fat" produces hormones and different substances that can cause destructive, constant impacts in the body, for example, harm to veins.

The DPP and different studies demonstrate that a great many individuals can bring down their danger for type 2 diabetes by rolling out way of life improvements and getting thinner. The DPP demonstrated that individuals with prediabetes—at high danger of creating type 2 diabetes—could forcefully bring down their danger by getting more fit through general physical movement and an eating regimen low in fat and calories. In 2009, a subsequent investigation of DPP members—the Diabetes Prevention Program Outcomes Study (DPPOS)— demonstrated that the advantages of weight reduction went on for no less than 10 years after the first study began.2

Perused more about the DPP, subsidized under National Institutes of Health (NIH) clinical trial number NCT00004992, and the DPPOS, financed under NIH clinical trial number NCT00038727 in Diabetes Prevention Program.

Insulin Resistance

Insulin resistance is a typical condition in individuals who are overweight or corpulent, have abundance stomach fat, and are not physically dynamic. Muscle, fat, and liver cells quit reacting legitimately to insulin, constraining the pancreas to repay by delivering additional insulin. For whatever length of time that beta cells can sufficiently deliver insulin, blood glucose levels stay in the ordinary reach. Be that as it may, when insulin generation vacillates because of beta cell brokenness, glucose levels rise, prompting prediabetes or diabetes.

Irregular Glucose Production by the Liver

In a few individuals with diabetes, an irregular increment in glucose generation by the liver additionally adds to high blood glucose levels. Ordinarily, the pancreas discharges the hormone glucagon when blood glucose and insulin levels are low. Glucagon animates the liver to create glucose and discharge it into the circulation system. In any case, when blood glucose and insulin levels are high after a supper, glucagon levels drop, and the liver stores overabundance glucose for some other time, when it is required. For reasons not totally comprehended, in numerous individuals with diabetes, glucagon levels stay higher than required. High glucagon levels cause the liver to deliver unneeded glucose, which adds to high blood glucose levels. Metformin, the most regularly utilized medication to treat type 2 diabetes, lessens glucose generation by the liver.

The Roles of Insulin and Glucagon in Normal Blood Glucose Regulation

A solid individual's body keeps blood glucose levels in an ordinary reach through a few complex systems. Insulin and glucagon, two hormones made in the pancreas, manage blood glucose levels:

Insulin, made by beta cells, brings down raised blood glucose levels.

Glucagon, made by alpha cells, raises low blood glucose levels.

At the point when blood glucose levels ascend after a supper, the pancreas discharges insulin into the blood.

Insulin muscles, fat, and liver cells ingest glucose from the circulation system, bringing down blood glucose levels.

Insulin invigorates the liver and muscle tissue to store overabundance glucose. The put away type of glucose is called glycogen.

Insulin likewise brings down blood glucose levels by lessening glucose generation in the liver.

At the point when blood glucose levels drop overnight or because of a skipped feast or substantial activity, the pancreas discharges glucagon into the blood. Glucagon flags the liver and muscle tissue to separate glycogen into glucose, which enters the circulation system and raises blood glucose levels. If that the body needs more glucose, glucagon invigorates the liver to make glucose from amino acids.

Drawing indicating two cutaway pictures of veins at the top and one cutaway picture of a vein at the base, each containing diverse measures of little circles speaking to glucose. The vein at the upper left with just a couple glucose circles is named Low blood glucose, and the vessel at the upper right, which contains numerous glucose circles, is named High blood glucose. The vessel at the base, with a middle of the road number of glucose circles, is named Normal blood glucose levels. A strong bolt focuses from the upper left vessel to a picture of a marked pancreas underneath. A sketched out bolt focuses from the upper right vessel to the pancreas picture underneath. Beneath the pancreas on the left is the name Glucagon discharged by pancreas and a strong bolt heading off to a drawing of the liver. Beneath the pancreas on the privilege is the mark Insulin discharged by pancreas and a laid out bolt setting off to a bunch of cells. Underneath the liver on the left side is the mark Liver discharges glucose into blood and a strong bolt encompassed by glucose hovers indicating the vein named Normal blood glucose levels. Beneath the group of cells on the privilege is the name Body's cells ingest glucose from blood and a plot bolt indicating the vein marked Normal blood glucose levels.

Insulin and glucagon control blood glucose levels.

Metabolic Syndrome

Metabolic disorder, additionally called insulin resistance disorder, alludes to a gathering of conditions regular in individuals with insulin resistance, including

higher than typical blood glucose levels greater waist size because of abundance stomach fat hypertension anomalous levels of cholesterol and triglycerides in the blood .

Individuals with metabolic disorder have an greater danger of creating type 2 diabetes and CVD. Numerous studies have found that way of life changes, for example, being physically dynamic and losing abundance weight, are the most ideal approaches to invert metabolic disorder, enhance the body's reaction to insulin, and decrease hazard for type 2 diabetes and CVD. Cell Signaling and Regulation

Cells impart through a mind boggling system of sub-atomic flagging pathways. For instance, on cell surfaces, insulin receptor particles catch, or tie, insulin atoms coursing in the circulation system. This association in the middle of insulin and its receptor prompts the biochemical signs that empower the cells to retain glucose from the blood and utilize it for vitality.

Issues in cell flagging frameworks can set off a chain response that prompts diabetes or different sicknesses. Numerous studies have concentrated on how insulin signals cells to impart and direct activity. Specialists have distinguished proteins and pathways that transmit the insulin flag and have mapped associations in the middle of insulin and body tissues, including the way insulin offers the liver control some assistance with blooding glucose levels. Analysts have likewise found that key flags additionally originate from fat cells, which create substances that cause irritation and insulin resistance.

This work holds the way to battling insulin resistance and diabetes. As researchers take in more about cell flagging frameworks included in glucose regulation, they will have more chances to create successful medicines.

Beta Cell Dysfunction
Researchers think beta cell brokenness is a key donor to type 2 diabetes. Beta cell debilitation can cause insufficient or anomalous examples of insulin discharge. Likewise, beta cells might be harmed by high blood glucose itself, a condition called glucose harmfulness.

Researchers have not decided the causes of beta cell brokenness as a rule. Single quality imperfections lead to particular types of diabetes called development onset diabetes of the youthful (MODY). The qualities included control insulin creation in the beta cells. Despite the fact that these types of diabetes are uncommon, they give pieces of information with reference to how beta cell capacity might be influenced by key administrative elements. Other quality variations are included in deciding the number and capacity of beta cells. Be that as it may, these variations represent just a little rate of type 2 diabetes cases. Hunger right on time in life is likewise being examined as a cause of beta cell brokenness. The metabolic environment of the creating hatchling might likewise make an inclination for diabetes sometime down the road.

Hazard Factors for Type 2 Diabetes

Individuals who have type 2 diabetes will probably have the accompanying attributes:

age 45 or more seasoned

overweight or large

physically idle

parent or kin with diabetes

family foundation that is African American, Alaska Native, American Indian, Asian American, Hispanic/Latino, or Pacific Islander American

history of bringing forth a child measuring more than 9 pounds

history of gestational diabetes

hypertension—140/90 or above—or being dealt with for hypertension

high-thickness lipoprotein (HDL), or great, cholesterol beneath 35 milligrams for each deciliter (mg/dL), or a triglyceride level above 250 mg/dL

polycystic ovary disorder, likewise called PCOS prediabetes—an A1C level of 5.7 to 6.4 percent; a fasting plasma glucose test consequence of 100–125 mg/dL, called disabled fasting glucose; or a 2-hour oral glucose resistance test aftereffect of 140–199, called debilitated glucose resilience acanthosis nigricans, a condition connected with insulin resistance, portrayed by a dull, smooth rash around the neck or armpits

History of CVD

The American Diabetes Association (ADA) prescribes that testing to recognize prediabetes and type 2 diabetes considered in grown-ups who are overweight or hefty and have one or more extra hazard components for diabetes. In grown-ups without these danger variables, testing ought to start at age 45.

2Diabetes Prevention Program Research Group. 10-year follow-up of diabetes occurrence and weight reduction in the Diabetes Prevention Program Outcomes Study.

What causes gestational diabetes?

Researchers accept gestational diabetes is caused by the hormonal changes and metabolic requests of pregnancy together with hereditary and ecological elements.

Insulin Resistance and Beta Cell Dysfunction

Hormones delivered by the placenta and other pregnancy-related variables add to insulin resistance, which happens in all ladies during late pregnancy. Insulin resistance builds the measure of insulin expected to control blood glucose levels. If that the pancreas can't create enough insulin because of beta cell brokenness, gestational diabetes happens.

Likewise with type 2 diabetes, overabundance weight is connected to gestational diabetes. Overweight or stout ladies are at especially high hazard for gestational diabetes because they begin pregnancy with a higher requirement for insulin because of insulin resistance. Intemperate weight pick up during pregnancy might likewise increment hazard.

Family History

Having a family history of diabetes is likewise a danger variable for gestational diabetes, recommending that qualities assume a part in its improvement. Hereditary qualities might likewise clarify why the confusion happens all the more every now and again in African Americans, American Indians, and Hispanics/Latinos. Numerous quality variations or blends of variations might expand a lady's danger for creating gestational diabetes. Considers have found a few quality variations connected with gestational diabetes, however these variations represent just a little portion of ladies with gestational diabetes.

Future Risk of Type 2 Diabetes

Because a lady's hormones as a rule come back to ordinary levels not long after in the wake of conceiving an offspring, gestational diabetes vanishes in most ladies after conveyance. In any case, ladies who have gestational diabetes will probably create gestational diabetes with future pregnancies and create type 2 diabetes.3 Women with gestational diabetes ought to be tried for relentless diabetes 6 to 12 weeks after conveyance and no less than at regular intervals from that point. Likewise, presentation to high glucose levels during growth builds a tyke's danger for getting to be overweight or hefty and for creating type 2 diabetes later on. The outcome might be a cycle of diabetes influencing various eras in a crew. For both mother and tyke, keeping up a solid body weight and being physically dynamic might avert type 2 diabetes.

Different Types and Causes of Diabetes

Different types of diabetes have an assortment of conceivable causes. Hereditary Mutations Affecting Beta Cells, Insulin, and Insulin Action Some generally unprecedented types of diabetes known as monogenic diabetes are caused by transformations, or changes, in a solitary quality. These transformations are typically acquired, yet here and there the quality change happens suddenly. A large portion of these quality transformations cause diabetes by diminishing beta cells' capacity to deliver insulin.

The most widely recognized types of monogenic diabetes are neonatal diabetes mellitus (NDM) and MODY. NDM happens in the initial 6 months of life. MODY is generally found during pre-adulthood or early adulthood however now and again is not analyzed until further down the road. More data about NDM and MODY is given in the NIDDK wellbeing theme, Monogenic Forms of Diabetes.

Other uncommon hereditary transformations can cause diabetes by harming the nature of insulin the body produces or by bringing on variations from the norm in insulin receptors.

Other Genetic Diseases

Diabetes happens in individuals with Down disorder, Klinefelter disorder, and Turner disorder at higher rates than the overall public. Researchers are exploring whether qualities that might incline individuals to hereditary disorders additionally incline them to diabetes. The hereditary issue cystic fibrosis and hemochromatosis are connected to diabetes. Cystic fibrosis creates anomalous thick bodily fluid, which obstructs the pancreas. The danger of diabetes increments with age in individuals with cystic fibrosis. Hemochromatosis causes the body to store an excessive amount of iron. If that the confusion is not treated, iron can develop in and harm the pancreas and different organs.

Harm to or Removal of the Pancreas

Pancreatitis, malignancy, and injury can all damage the pancreatic beta cells or debilitate insulin generation, hence bringing about diabetes. If that the harmed pancreas is uprooted, diabetes will happen because of the loss of the beta cells. Endocrine Diseases Endocrine illnesses influence organs that deliver hormones. Cushing's disorder and acromegaly are illustrations of hormonal issue that can cause prediabetes and diabetes by affecting insulin resistance. Cushing's disorder is set apart by unreasonable creation of cortisol—some of the time called the "anxiety hormone." Acromegaly happens when the body delivers an excessive amount of development hormone. Glucagonoma, an uncommon tumor of the pancreas, can likewise cause diabetes. The tumor causes the body to deliver a lot of glucagon. Hyperthyroidism, a confusion that happens when the thyroid organ delivers an excess of thyroid hormone, can likewise cause lifted blood glucose levels.

Immune system Disorders

Uncommon disarranges described by antibodies that upset insulin activity can prompt diabetes. This sort of diabetes is frequently connected with other immune system issue, for example, lupus erythematosus. Another uncommon immune system issue called firm man disorder is connected with antibodies that assault the beta cells, like type 1 diabetes.

Solutions and Chemical Toxins

A few solutions, for example, nicotinic corrosive and certain types of diuretics, hostile to seizure drugs, psychiatric medications, and medications to treat human immunodeficiency infection (HIV), can disable beta cells or disturb insulin activity. Pentduringine, a medication endorsed to treat a type of pneumonia, can build the danger of pancreatitis, beta cell harm, and diabetes. Likewise, glucocorticoids—steroid hormones that are artificially like actually created cortisol—might impede insulin activity. Glucocorticoids are utilized to regard incendiary sicknesses, for example, rheumatoid joint pain, asthma, lupus, and ulcerative colitis.

Numerous concoction poisons can harm or demolish beta cells in creatures, however just a couple have been connected to diabetes in people. For instance, dioxin—a contaminant of the herbicide Agent Orange, utilized during the Vietnam War—might be connected to the advancement of type 2 diabetes. In 2000, in view of a report from the Institute of Medicine, the U.S. Branch of Veterans Affairs (VA) added diabetes to the rundown of conditions for which Vietnam veterans are qualified for incapacity remuneration. Likewise, a compound in a rodent toxic substance no more being used has been appeared to cause diabetes if ingested. A few studies recommend a high admission of nitrogen-containing chemicals, for example, nitrates and nitrites may build the danger of diabetes. Arsenic has additionally been concentrated on for conceivable connections to diabetes.

Lipodystrophy

Lipodystrophy is a condition in which fat tissue is lost or redistributed in the body. The condition is connected with insulin resistance and type 2 diabetes. Diabetes is an unpredictable gathering of ailments with an assortment of causes. Researchers trust qualities and ecological elements collaborate to cause diabetes much of the time. Individuals with diabetes have high blood glucose, additionally called high glucose or hyperglycemia. Diabetes creates when the body doesn't make enough insulin or is not ready to utilize insulin adequately, or both.

Insulin is a hormone made by beta cells in the pancreas. Insulin offers cells all through the body some assistance with absorbing and utilize glucose for vitality. If that the body does not sufficiently deliver insulin or can't utilize insulin viably, glucose develops in the blood as opposed to being consumed by cells in the body, and the body is famished of vitality.

Prediabetes is a condition in which blood glucose levels or A1C levels are higher than ordinary yet not sufficiently high to be analyzed as diabetes. Individuals with prediabetes can significantly diminish their danger of losing so as to create diabetes weight and expanding physical action.

The two primary types of diabetes are type 1 diabetes and type 2 diabetes. Gestational diabetes is a third type of diabetes that grows just during pregnancy. Type 1 diabetes is caused by an absence of insulin because of the demolition of insulin-creating beta cells. In type 1 diabetes—an immune system illness—the body's invulnerable framework assaults and decimates the beta cells. Type 2 diabetes—the most widely recognized type of diabetes—is caused by a blend of variables, including insulin resistance, a condition in which the body's muscle, fat, and liver cells don't utilize insulin viably. Type 2 diabetes creates when the body can no more sufficiently deliver insulin to make up for the disabled capacity to utilize insulin.

Researchers accept gestational diabetes is caused by the hormonal changes and metabolic requests of pregnancy together with hereditary and natural elements. Hazard variables for gestational diabetes incorporate being overweight and having a family history of diabetes. Monogenic types of diabetes are generally exceptional and are caused by transformations in single qualities that breaking point insulin creation, quality, or activity in the body. Different types of diabetes are caused by sicknesses and wounds that harm the pancreas; certain concoction poisons and solutions; contaminations; and different conditions.

To comprehend diabetes, first you should see how glucose is typically handled in the body.

How insulin functions

Insulin is a hormone that originates from an organ arranged behind and underneath the stomach (pancreas).

The pancreas secretes insulin into the circulatory system.

The insulin flows, empowering sugar to enter your phones.

Insulin brings down the measure of sugar in your circulatory system.

As your glucose level drops, so does the discharge of insulin from your pancreas.

The role of glucose

Glucose — a sugar — is a wellspring of vitality for the phones that make up muscles and different tissues. Glucose originates from two noteworthy sources: nourishment and your liver. Sugar is consumed into the circulation system, where it enters cells with the assistance of insulin. Your liver stores and makes glucose. At the point when your glucose levels are low, for example, when you haven't eaten in a while, the liver separates put away glycogen into glucose to keep your glucose level inside of an ordinary reach.

Causes of type 1 diabetes

The careful cause of type 1 diabetes is obscure. What is known is that your resistant framework — which ordinarily battles destructive microscopic organisms or infections — assaults and wrecks your insulin-creating cells in the pancreas. This abandons you with next to zero insulin. Rather than being transported into your cells, sugar develops in your circulatory system. Type 1 is thought to be caused by a blend of hereditary helplessness and natural elements, however precisely what a number of those components are is still vague.

Causes of prediabetes and type 2 diabetes

In prediabetes — which can prompt type 2 diabetes — and in type 2 diabetes, your cells get to be impervious to the activity of insulin, and your pancreas can't make enough insulin to beat this resistance. Rather than moving into your cells where it's required for vitality, sugar develops in your circulatory system. Precisely why this happens is indeterminate, in spite of the fact that it's trusted that hereditary and natural elements assume a part in the advancement of type 2 diabetes. Being overweight is emphatically connected to the advancement of type 2 diabetes, yet not everybody with type 2 is overweight.

Causes of gestational diabetes

During pregnancy, the placenta produces hormones to maintain your pregnancy. These hormones make your cells more impervious to insulin. Typically, your pancreas reacts by delivering enough additional insulin to defeat this resistance. Be that as it may, here and there your pancreas can't keep up. At the point when this happens, too little glucose gets into your cells and an excess of stays in your blood, bringing about gestation.

Diabetes causes differ contingent upon your hereditary cosmetics, family history, ethnicity, wellbeing and natural components. The reason there is no characterized diabetes cause is because the causes of diabetes shift contingent upon the individual and the type. Case in point; the causes of type 1 diabetes change extensively from the causes of gestational diabetes. Additionally, the causes of type 2 diabetes are unmistakable from the causes of type 1 diabetes.

Causes of type 1 diabetes

Type 1 diabetes causes

Type 1 diabetes is caused by the insusceptible framework devastating the cells in the pancreas that make insulin. This causes diabetes by leaving the body without enough insulin to work regularly.

This is called an immune system response, or immune system cause, because the body is assaulting itself. There is no particular diabetes causes, yet the accompanying triggers might be included:

Viral or bacterial infection

Substance poisons inside of nourishment

Unidentified part bringing about immune system response

Hidden hereditary aura might likewise be a type 1 diabetes cause.

Type 2 diabetes causes

Type 2 diabetes causes are generally multifactorial - more than one diabetes cause is included. Regularly, the most overpowering component is a family history of type 2 diabetes.

There are an assortment of danger elements for type 2 diabetes, any or all of which expand the odds of building up the condition.

These include:

Heftiness

Carrying on with a sedentary way of life

 ageing

Awful eating regimen

Other type 2 diabetes causes, for example, pregnancy or ailment can be type 2 diabetes hazard variables.

Point by point causes of diabetes are still not all that surely knew, on the other hand, various components have been distinguished as expanding the odds of creating distinctive types of diabetes.

Gestational diabetes

Type 1 diabetes is an auto-insusceptible illness, implying that the body's safe framework assaults its body's own cells. In type 1 diabetes, the insulin creating cells are relentlessly executed off by the resistant framework. Hereditary elements are known not a section with type 1 diabetes frequently running in families. Another variable that is by all accounts having an effect on everything is that type 1 diabetes is more regular in nations further from the equator, recommending that vitamin D might have impact.

With the pervasiveness of type 2 diabetes expanding so rapidly, there has been much examination around the causes of this metabolic condition. Hereditary qualities is one region of center with particular qualities seeming to improve the probability of type 2 diabetes creating.

There are clear connections to ethnicity also with individuals of South Asian, Middle Eastern and African-Caribbean plummet at a higher danger of type 2 diabetes. Eating regimen is broadly accepted to be a variable in type 2 diabetes, on the other hand, there is some difference as to which parts of our eating routine could be mindful.

Soaked and trans fats, prepared sustenances and over the top starch having all been mooted as could reasonably be expected causal variables. Gestational diabetes is a type of diabetes that particularly goes ahead during pregnancy. During the second and third trimesters of pregnancy, with prerequisites for insulin officially developing, hormones discharged by the placenta can prompt insulin being less successful. If that the mother's body battles to sufficiently deliver insulin, glucose levels can rise bringing about gestational diabetes.

Causes of Gestational diabetes

The causes of diabetes in pregnancy otherwise called gestational diabetes stay obscure. On the other hand, there are various danger elements that expand the odds of adding to this condition:

Family history of gestational diabetes

Overweight or hefty

Experience the ill effects of polycystic ovary disorder

Have had a child weighing more than 9lb .Causes of gestational diabetes might likewise be identified with ethnicity - some ethnic gatherings have a higher danger of gestational diabetes.

Different diabetes causes

There are an assortment of other potential diabetes causes. These incorporate the accompanying:

Pancreatitis or pancreatectomy as a cause of diabetes. Pancreatitis is known not the danger of creating diabetes, just like a pancreatectomy. Polycystic Ovary Syndrome (PCOS). One of the underlying drivers of PCOS is heftiness connected insulin resistance, which might likewise expand the danger of pre-diabetes and type 2 diabetes.

Cushing's disease

This disorder expands creation of the cortisol hormone, which serves to greater blood glucose levels. An excess of cortisol can cause diabetes. Glucagonoma. Patients with glucagonoma might encounter diabetes because of an absence of balance between levels of insulin creation and glucagon generation.

Steroid actuated diabetes (steroid diabetes) is an uncommon type of diabetes that happens because of delayed utilization of glucocorticoid treatment.

Causes for type 2 diabetes

Type 2 diabetes happens when the pancreas doesn't create enough insulin to keep up a typical blood glucose level, or the body can't utilize the insulin that is delivered – known as insulin resistance. The pancreas (a vast organ behind the stomach) delivers the hormone insulin, which moves glucose from your blood into your cells, where it's changed over into vitality. In type 2 diabetes, there are a few causes why the pancreas doesn't sufficiently deliver insulin.

Hazardous elements for type 2 diabetes

Four of the fundamental danger elements for creating type 2 diabetes are:

age – being beyond 40 25 years old (25 for south Asian individuals)

Genetic characteristics
having a nearby relative with the condition (guardian, sibling or sister)

Being overweight
being overweight or fat

ethnicity –
being of south Asian, Chinese, African-Caribbean or dark African source (regardless of the possibility that you were conceived in the UK)

Your danger of creating type 2 diabetes increments with age. This might be on the grounds that individuals tend to put on weight and practice less as they get more seasoned. Eating so as to keep up a sound weight a solid, adjusted eating routine and practicing consistently are methods for averting and overseeing diabetes. White individuals beyond 40 a years old an greater danger of creating type 2 diabetes. Individuals of south Asian, Chinese, African-Caribbean and dark African drop have an greater danger of creating type 2 diabetes at a much prior age. Be that as it may, regardless of expanding age being a danger variable for type 2 diabetes, over late years more youthful individuals from every ethnic gathering have been adding to the condition.

It's additionally turning out to be more regular for youngsters, at times as youthful as seven, to create type 2 diabetes.

Genetic characteristics

Hereditary qualities is one of the principle hazard components for type 2 diabetes. Your danger of building up the condition is greater if that you have a nearby relative –, for example, a guardian, sibling or sister – who has the condition. The closer the relative, the more noteworthy the danger. A kid who has a guardian with type 2 diabetes has around an one in three possibility of additionally creating it (see beneath).

Being overweight or stout

Will probably create type 2 diabetes in case you're overweight or corpulent (with a body mass record (BMI) of 30 or more). Specifically, fat around your tummy (guts) builds your danger. This is on the grounds that it discharges chemicals that can agitate the body's cardiovascular and metabolic frameworks.

This builds your danger of adding to various genuine conditions, including coronary illness, stroke and a few types of tumor. Measuring your waist is a speedy method for evaluating your diabetes hazard. This is a measure of stomach weight, which is an especially high-hazard type of heftiness.

Ladies have a higher danger of creating type 2 diabetes if their waist measures 80cm (31.5 inches) or more. Asian men with a waist size of 89cm (35 inches) or over have a higher danger, as do white or dark men with a waist size of 94cm (37 inches) or over. Utilize the BMI adding machine to see whether you're a solid weight for your stature.

Practicing routinely and decreasing your body weight by around 5% could lessen your danger of getting diabetes by more than half.

Ethnicity

Individuals of south Asian, Chinese, African-Caribbean and dark African will probably create type 2 diabetes. Type 2 diabetes is up to six times more regular in south Asian groups than in the general UK populace, and it's three times more basic among individuals of African and African-Caribbean root.

Individuals of south Asian and African-Caribbean starting point likewise have an greater danger of creating confusions of diabetes, for example, coronary illness, at a more youthful age than whatever remains of the populace.

Different dangers

Your danger of creating type 2 diabetes is additionally greater if your blood glucose level is higher than ordinary, yet not yet sufficiently high to be determined to have diabetes. This is here and there called "pre-diabetes" – specialists some of the time call it debilitated fasting glycaemia (IFG) or weakened glucose resistance (IGT). Pre-diabetes can advance to type 2 diabetes if that you don't make safeguard strides, for example, rolling out way of life improvements. These incorporate eating soundly, shedding pounds (in case you're overweight) and taking a lot of standard activity.

Ladies who have had gestational diabetes during pregnancy likewise have a more serious danger of creating diabetes.

Chapter 4

Some facts about diabetes

Type 2 diabetes is the most well-known type of diabetes. Around 90 to 95% of individuals with diabetes have type 2 diabetes.

Being overweight (BMI more noteworthy than 25) builds your danger of creating type 2 diabetes. There's a hereditary transformation included in type 2 diabetes, in spite of the fact that analysts haven't possessed the capacity to pinpoint the careful change. You should have a hereditary change with a specific end goal to create type 2—not everybody can get it. If you have a family history, you are at higher danger.

Numerous individuals are overweight when they're determined to have type 2 diabetes. On the other hand, you don't need to be overweight to create it.

Type 2 used to be called "grown-up onset diabetes" since it was analyzed mostly in more established individuals. Today, however, more youngsters around the globe are being determined to have type 2, so type 2 is the more basic name now.

A great many people with type 2 diabetes are insulin safe, implying that their bodies don't utilize insulin legitimately. They make all that could possibly be needed of it, yet their cells are impervious to it and don't know how to utilize it legitimately.

A few individuals with type 2 diabetes don't sufficiently deliver insulin.

Type 2 diabetes can more often than not be overseen well with a blend of more advantageous dinner arrangement decisions, physical movement, and oral solutions. A few individuals might need to take insulin so as to improve blood glucose control.

Did you know these 10 truths about diabetes?

Around 33% surprisingly with diabetes don't know they have the malady.

Type 2 diabetes frequently does not have any side effects.

Just around five percent surprisingly with diabetes have type 1 diabetes.

If you are at danger, type 2 diabetes can be counteracted with moderate weight reduction (10–15 pounds) and 30 minutes of moderate physical action, (for example, lively strolling) every day.

A feast arrangement for a man with diabetes isn't altogether different than that which is suggested for individuals without diabetes.

Diabetes is the main source of visual deficiency in working-age grown-ups.

Individuals with diabetes are twice as liable to create coronary illness than somebody without diabetes.

Great control of diabetes significantly lessens the danger of creating entanglements and keeps intricacies from deteriorating.

Bariatric surgery can lessen the side effects of diabetes in hefty individuals.

Diabetes costs $174 billion every year, incorporating $116 billion in direct restorative costs.

Type 2 diabetes, which is generally activated by stoutness, has gotten a great deal of press since it used to strike just grown-ups and is currently being analyzed in children as youthful as 6, says Dr. Laffel. Disturbing as that may be, a more noteworthy number of children get type 1, an immune system sickness that has been rising 4 percent a year since the 1970s - particularly in youthful children. Just 3,700 kids are determined to have type 2 consistently contrasted and 15,000 who create type 1, as per a substantial study that gives the initially itemized take a gander at diabetes in U.S. kids. From numerous points of view, the two types of diabetes are altogether different. In type 1, which has no known reason, the insusceptible framework erroneously annihilates sound cells in the pancreas that create insulin, the hormone that offers the body some assistance with getting vitality from sustenance. To compensate for the setback, youngsters commonly require infusions of insulin a few times each day. In type 2, the pancreas typically makes a lot of insulin (in any event at first), however cells all through the body experience difficulty utilizing it - a condition known as insulin resistance. Be that as it may, regardless of what the type, diabetes causes high glucose levels when glucose from sustenance - what might as well be called gas for an auto - develops in light of the fact that it can't get into cells without insulin. After some time, overabundance glucose can harm organs and tissues all through the body.

Reality: White Children Are at the Highest Risk

Numerous individuals have heard that diabetes is to a greater degree a danger to minorities, yet around 71 percent of all kids who have the sickness are white, gauge analysts in the historic point SEARCH for Diabetes in Youth Study. "Type 1 diabetes, which is much more basic than type 2, happens at higher rates in whites," says Dana Dabelea, MD, PhD, partner educator of medication in the division of preventive solution and biometrics at the University of Colorado Denver Health Sciences Center. In spite of the fact that type 2 occurs all the more oftentimes in minorities - including African-Americans and Hispanics - their general danger of getting diabetes is much lower.

Reality: Diabetes Isn't Caused by Eating Too Much Sugar

While type 2 is regularly identified with being overweight, sugar has no more prominent effect on glucose levels in the blood than different types of starches such as rice and potatoes. Specialists are worried about sugar for the most part since it's found in swelling nourishments like treats and frozen yogurt that youngsters love. "Youngsters who are at high danger of type 2 diabetes don't just eat an excessive amount of sugar, they eat a lot of everything," says Dr. Dabelea. Kids who as of now have diabetes need to cutoff desserts and basic carbs so as to keep their glucose in line, however even a kid with type 1 diabetes can eat a brownie once in a while the length of she takes additional insulin to offer her body some assistance with processing the sugar, says M.

Jennifer Abuzzahab, MD, an endocrinologist at Children's Hospitals and Clinics of Minnesota, in St. Paul.

Reality: Kids with Diabetes Won't Necessarily Need Insulin Shots

Numerous youngsters who have type 2 diabetes can get their glucose levels under control just by eating better, getting more fit, and practicing consistently, which can offer insulin some assistance with working all the more viably. If these lifestyle changes aren't sufficient, they can likewise take oral solutions like metformin. Be that as it may, even children who need to take insulin - all youngsters with type 1 and half of those with type 2 - don't have to face shots consistently. "About a large portion of the children in our center utilize a pump," says Dr. Abuzzahab. This pager-like gadget, which is cut to a waistband or strapped to the middle, is customized to direct a consistent stream of insulin through a port in the skin. After a supper or nibble, when rising glucose levels make interest for more insulin, a kid can get an additional measurement by simply pushing a catch.

Reality: Even If a Child with Diabetes Feels Healthy, She's Still at Risk for Serious Complications

Keeping glucose levels ordinary all through life is the way to keeping an assortment of issues. Left uncorrected, diabetes can prompt heart assault, cirrhosis of the liver, visual deficiency, removal of appendages influenced by poor flow, and kidney disappointment that requires lifelong dialysis. Luckily, there's an ideal opportunity to keep these desperate conditions while kids are still youthful: It takes around five to 10 years for ineffectively controlled glucose to create any real inconveniences, as per specialists. Genuine difficulties are not unavoidable, says Dr. Abuzzahab. "They're all identified with poor glucose control, and most children can diminish their danger with the right treatment."

Could Environment Be a Factor in Childhood Diabetes?

Rates of type 1 diabetes have been consistently climbing around the world. "While early youth is still the most widely recognized time of onset, a few kids are being analyzed even before their first birthday," says Dr. Laffel. Despite the fact that children who create type 1 are thought to have some kind of hereditary inclination to a breaking down invulnerable framework, most don't have a nearby relative with the condition. The explanation behind the ascent is a riddle, however analysts are investigating three ecological components.

Great Cleanliness Thanks to enhanced cleanliness, kids don't experience the same number of germs today, which might meddle with ordinary improvement of the safe framework.

Weight Gain In children whose insulin-creating cells have as of now begun breaking down, abundance weight might quicken the improvement of out and out diabetes.

Early Solids Feeding oat before 3 months to an infant who is at higher danger for type 1 might be connected to setting off the resistant framework to erroneously assault his pancreas.

"Diabetes" is Greek for "siphon," which alludes to the abundant pee of uncontrolled diabetes. "Mellitus" is Latin for "nectar" or "sweet," a name included when doctors found that the pee from individuals with diabetes is sweet with glucose.Researchers foresee that there might be 30 million new instances of diabetes in China alone by 2025.a

The soonest recorded notice of an illness that can be perceived as diabetes is found in the Ebers papyrus (1500 B.C.), which incorporates bearings for a few blends that could "evacuate the pee, which runs too often."

The name "diabetes" is credited to the acclaimed Greek doctor Aretaeus of Cappadocia who honed in the first century A.D. He trusted that diabetes was brought about by snakebite.a

William Cullen (1710-1790), a teacher of science and pharmaceutical in Scotland, is in charge of including the expression "mellitus" ("sweet" or "nectar like") to the word diabetes.a

In 1889, Oskar Minkowski (1858-191931) found the connection in the middle of diabetes and the pancreas (dish - "all" + kreas - "substance) when a puppy from which he evacuated the pancreas created diabetes.a

Insulin was begat from the Latin insula ("island") in light of the fact that the hormone is emitted by the Islets of Langerhans in the pancreas.i

Prior to the revelation of insulin, specialists once in a while worked on diabetic patients with gangrene in light of the fact that the patients ordinarily would not recuperate and would definitely pass on. Now and again, a range of gangrene would "auto-cut off," which means it would become scarce and fall off.a

Prior to the disclosure of insulin in 1921, doctors would frequently put their patients on starvation or semi-starvation diets, prescribing they eat just nourishments, for example, oatmeal.

Weight

Weight has prompted a sensational increment in Type 2 diabetes

Around 90% of individuals with Type 2 diabetes are obese.c

In 1996, a 16-year-old young lady with diabetes kicked the bucket at her home in Altoona, Pennsylvania, since her guardians declined to give her medication and depended on supplication to God. Her guardians were accused of manslaughter.a

A few scientists have discovered connections between the onset of Type 1 diabetes and the contracting of an infection, particularly the mumps or Coxsacki virus.a

African-Americans and Hispanics have a much higher rate of Type 2 diabetes than whites. There are 74 cases for each 1,000 for African-Americans, 61 cases for Hispanics, and 36 cases for whites.a

The demise rate among African-Americans with diabetes is 27% higher than among whites with diabetes. Reasons incorporate innate, financial issues, higher stoutness rates, and absence of accessible medical coverage or protection coverage.a

Roughly one in three African-American ladies between the ages of 65-74 have diabetes.a

A few studies have shown that people with diabetes are at much more serious danger for adding to Alzheimer's ailment and different types of dementia than are non-diabetics, however the reasons are unknown.a

There are around 86,000 lower-appendage removals on diabetics in the United States every year. Rates of removal were higher among men than ladies and higher among African-Americans than whites. Specialists accept almost 50% of all removals could have been anticipated with proper examinations and education.a

Diabetes has been accounted for in steeds, ferrets, and ground squirrels. In situations where creatures are generously bolstered, diabetes has been accounted for in dolphins, foxes, and even a hippopotamus.

a visual impairment

Diabetes is a main source of visual impairment in American grown-ups

Diabetes is the primary driver of visual deficiency in people matured 20-74 in the United States. Specialists underscore that early location and treatment could counteract up to 90% of instances of visual deficiency that are identified with diabetes.h

Despite the fact that coronary illness has dropped among non-diabetic ladies by 27%, it has really greater by 23% for ladies with diabetes.g

Surely understood individuals with diabetes incorporate Mary Tyler Moore, Jerry Mathers (Leave it to Beaver), and Jerry Garcia of The Grateful Dead. The late Carroll O'Conner from the TV demonstrate All in the Family had diabetes and had his toe excised in 2000.a

Olympic swimmer Gary Hall Jr. has Type 1 diabetes. When he was analyzed, his doctor instructed him to surrender swimming. He changed specialists, kept preparing, and therefore won a gold medal.a

White youngsters have a more serious danger of creating Type 1 diabetes than offspring of different races, however the occurrence of the illness changes incredibly from nation to nation. Hazard elements incorporate being sick in right on time early stages, having a more established mother, having a mother with Type 1 diabetes, having a mother who had preeclampsia during pregnancy, and having a high conception weight.

Those with diabetes will probably create carpal passage disorder and tarsal passage syndrome.

Those with diabetes, especially youthful young ladies with Type 1 diabetes, might be at greater danger of creating dietary issues. Some juvenile young ladies intentionally withhold their insulin to lose weight.

Around 11% of all Americans matured 65-74 have diabetes. Around 20% of those more than 75 years of age have diabetes, and about portion of them are uninformed they have the disease.a

By Centers for Disease Control and Prevention (CDC), diabetes is the 6th driving reason for death in the United States.d

Men with diabetes are at a more serious danger for erectile brokenness (ED) than non-diabetic men. Roughly 50-60% of men with diabetes beyond 50 years old have issues with ED. Also, ED turns into an issue for diabetic men around 10 to 15 years sooner than a non-diabetic man.

apple-molded body

An apple-molded body, or abundance stomach fat, is a danger element for Type 2 diabetes

People with an "apple" body shape are at more serious danger for diabetes than are those with "pear" body shapes.b

Ladies with diabetes will probably create vaginal contaminations than are non-diabetics in view of their hoisted glucose levels.h

People who have acquired other hereditary disorders (Down's disorder, myotonic disorder, Turner's disorder) are likewise at danger of creating diabetes.

Diabetics have a higher danger of gingivitis than non-diabetics, which might prompt bone and tooth misfortune. On the other hand, just about portion of Hispanics with diabetes routinely visit a dental practitioner contrasted with 58% of African-Americans and 70% of non-Hispanic whites with diabetes.

Breathed in insulin is a rising twenty-first century choice for individuals with Type 1 diabetes. Organizations are likewise taking a shot at an insulin tablet that can be given under the tongue.h

While Hispanics have a higher rate of Type 2 diabetes than non-Hispanic whites, they regularly live more than non-Hispanic whites on kidney dialysis.

People with diabetes are more vulnerable to inconveniences of influenza and pneumonia and are six times more inclined to be hospitalized for these issues than non-diabetics. By Centers for Disease Control, 10,000-30,000 individuals with diabetes bite the dust every year from influenza and pneumonia.

Specialists report that diabetes diminishes life hope by five to 10 years.

Men have a higher danger of death from diabetes than women.g

Specialists recommend that normal glucose levels can be higher for diabetic young ladies with menstrual difficulties. Moreover, young ladies with menstrual issues likewise had a higher rate of clinic affirmations for diabetic ketoacidosis (DKA). By Department of Veterans Affairs, diabetes is more pervasive among military veterans than in the all inclusive community. Around 16% of military veterans (or around 500,000) have diabetes, contrasted with 6% of the general U.S. public.a

cereal

The solvent fiber in oats controls blood glucose levels. A Harvard study demonstrated that eating one serving of cooked cereal two to four times each week was connected to a 16% diminishment in the danger of creating Type 2 diabetes. One serving five or six times each week was connected to a 39% lessening in risk.a

Diabetes mellitus is a general name that envelops a few types of diabetes, including Type 1, Type 2, gestational, and varieties, for example, development onset diabetes in the youthful (MODY) and inert immune system diabetes of adulthood (LADA). What they all have in like manner is the powerlessness to self-control levels of blood glucose (cell fuel) in the body.

Roughly 17 million U.S. inhabitants have been determined to have diabetes, which is almost 10% of the evaluated 170 million individuals experiencing diabetes worldwide.d

Diabetes insipidus (water diabetes) is a condition totally different from diabetes mellitus. Diabetes insipidus is portrayed by an issue with the kidneys in which the kidneys can't focus pee satisfactorily because of an insufficiency in the antidiuretic hormone (ADH).Antiquated specialists would test for diabetes by tasting the pee of an associated sufferer with diabetes. Sweet pee is high in glucose, recommending the vicinity of diabetes.

Certain sicknesses, for example, cystic fibrosis, pancreatitis, hemochromatosis, and Cushing's disorder—might make pancreatic beta cell pulverization that leads diabetes.

Clinical exploration found that infants who breastfeed no less than three months had a lower frequency of Type 1 diabetes and might be less inclined to end up corpulent as adults.

An expected 16 million Americans have pre-diabetes, and large portions of them are uninformed of their condition.

Overweight people are more inclined to create diabetes since more fat requires more insulin, fat cells discharge free unsaturated fats which meddle with glucose digestion system, and overweight individuals have less accessible insulin receptors.

Constricting so as to smoke can expand diabetes hazard veins, raising circulatory strain, and animating the arrival of catecholamines (battle or-flight hormones), which advance insulin resistance.

Gestational diabetes happens in around 200,000 or 7% of U.S. pregnancies annually.

cash

U.S. diabetes expenses are about $200 billion yearly

Diabetes in the United States alone expenses $200 billion every year. This figure incorporates direct therapeutic costs, for example, insulin, removals, and hospitalizations and additionally aberrant costs, for example, lost efficiency, early retirement, and disability.d

Insulin in the 1920s was at first separated from the pancreas of a (cow-like) or pig (porcine). Today's insulins are made in the lab, refined from microscopic organisms and yeast through recombinant DNA.a

The human body is outfitted with 60,000 miles of veins and set up with 100,000 miles of nerve filaments. Diabetes frequently obstructs the cardiovascular framework and stifles nerves, bringing about 80% of passings among patients with diabetes.h

In ladies, diabetes sways estrogen levels, menstrual and ovulation cycles, and sexual desire.g

Specialists found that at regular intervals spent sitting in front of the TV was connected with a 14% expansion in diabetes risk.h

There are around 1 million individuals in the United States with Type 1 diabetes, yet just 2,000 contributor pancreases are accessible every year for transplants.

People with diabetes will probably kick the bucket from a heart assault than the individuals who don't have diabetes.Twelve million men (11.2% of all men 20 years and more established) and 11.5 million ladies (10.2% of all ladies 20 years and more seasoned) have diabetes in the U.S.d

Diabetes is the main source of kidney disappointment, representing 44% of new cases in 2005.d

Around 60-70% of individuals with diabetes have gentle to extreme types of sensory system damage.

Chapter 5

Traditional western treatments

Management of type 2 diabetes incorporates:

Adhering to a good diet

Consistent activity

diabetes drug or insulin treatment

Glucose monitoring

These strides will keep your glucose level closer to typical, which can postpone or anticipate confusions.

Adhering to a good diet

In spite of well known recognition, there's no particular diabetes diet. Be that as it may, it's critical to fixate your eating regimen on these high-fiber, low-fat nourishments:

Low glycemic list sustenances additionally might be useful. The glycemic record is a measure of how rapidly a nourishment causes an ascent in your glucose. Sustenances with a high glycemic list raise your glucose rapidly. Low glycemic list nourishments might offer you some assistance with achieving a more steady glucose. Sustenances with a low glycemic file commonly are nourishments that are higher in fiber.

An enrolled dietitian can offer you some assistance with putting together a feast plan that fits your wellbeing objectives, nourishment inclinations and way of life. He or she can likewise show you how to screen your starch allow and let you think about what number of sugars you have to eat with your suppers and snacks to keep your glucose levels more steady.

Exercise

Everybody needs customary vigorous work out, and individuals who have type 2 diabetes are no special case. Get your specialist's OK before you begin an activity program. At that point pick exercises you appreciate, for example, strolling, swimming and biking. What's most essential is making physical movement some portion of your every day schedule.

Go for no less than 30 minutes of high-impact exercise five days of the week. Extending and quality preparing activities are critical, as well. If that you haven't been dynamic for some time, begin gradually and develop continuously.

A mix of activities — oxygen consuming activities, for example, strolling or moving on most days, joined with resistance preparing, for example, weightlifting or yoga twice per week — regularly controls glucose more successfully than either type of activity alone.

Keep in mind that physical action brings down glucose. Check your glucose level before any movement. You may need to eat a nibble before practicing to avert low glucose if that you take diabetes pharmaceuticals that lower your glucose.

Monitoring your glucose

Contingent upon your treatment arrangement, you might need to check and record your glucose level from time to time or, in case you're on insulin, different times each day. Ask your specialist how regularly he or she needs you to check your glucose. Watchful checking is the best way to ensure that your glucose level stays inside of your objective reach.

Here and there, glucose levels can be erratic. With assistance from your diabetes treatment group, you'll figure out how your glucose level changes because of nourishment, activity, liquor, disease and medicine.

Diabetes medicines and insulin treatment

A few individuals who have type 2 diabetes can accomplish their objective glucose levels with eating regimen and practice alone, yet numerous likewise require diabetes meds or insulin treatment. The choice about which drugs are best relies on upon numerous components, including your glucose level and whatever other wellbeing issues you have. Your specialist may even consolidate drugs from various classes to offer you some assistance with controlling your glucose in a few unique ways.

Cases of conceivable medications for type 2 diabetes include:

Metformin
(Glucophage, Glumetza, others). For the most part, metformin is the first solution endorsed for type 2 diabetes. It works by enhancing the affectability of your body tissues to insulin so that your body utilizes insulin all the more successfully.

Metformin likewise brings down glucose generation in the liver. Metformin may not bring down glucose enough all alone. Your specialist will likewise suggest way of life changes, for example, getting in shape and turning out to be more dynamic.

Queasiness and looseness of the bowels are conceivable reactions of metformin. These reactions typically leave as your body gets used to the solution. If that metformin and ways of life changes aren't sufficient to control your glucose level, other oral or infused pharmaceuticals can be included.

Sulfonylureas.
These solutions offer your body some assistance with secreting more insulin. Samples of pharmaceuticals in this class incorporate glyburide (DiaBeta, Glynase), glipizide (Glucotrol) and glimepiride (Amaryl). Conceivable symptoms incorporate low glucose and weight pick up.

Meglitinides.

These drugs work like sulfonylureas by fortifying the pancreas to emit more insulin, yet they're speedier acting, and the length of time of their impact in the body is shorter. They likewise have a danger of bringing about low glucose, however this danger is lower than with sulfonylureas.

Weight addition is a probability with this class of meds too. Cases incorporate repaglinide (Prandin) and nateglinide (Starlix).

Thiazolidinediones.

Like metformin, these solutions make the body's tissues more touchy to insulin. This class of medicines has been connected to weight pick up and other more-genuine symptoms, for example, an greater danger of heart disappointment and breaks. Because of these dangers, these solutions for the most part aren't a first-decision treatment.

Rosiglitazone

(Avandia) and pioglitazone (Actos) are illustrations of thiazolidinediones.

DPP-4 inhibitors.

These solutions decrease glucose levels, yet have a tendency to have an unobtrusive impact. They don't cause weight pick up. Illustrations of these pharmaceuticals are sitagliptin (Januvia), saxagliptin (Onglyza) and linagliptin (Tradjenta).

GLP-1 receptor agonists.
These solutions moderate processing and bring down glucose levels, however not as much as sulfonylureas. Their utilization is frequently connected with some weight reduction. This class of solutions isn't suggested for use without anyone else.

Exenatide (Byetta)
and liraglutide (Victoza) are samples of GLP-1 receptor agonists. Conceivable symptoms incorporate sickness and an greater danger of pancreatitis.

SGLT2 inhibitors.
These are the most up to date diabetes drugs available. They work by keeping the kidneys from reabsorbing sugar into the blood. Rather, the sugar is discharged in the pee.

Samples incorporate canagliflozin (Invokana) and dapagliflozin (Farxiga). Symptoms might incorporate yeast diseases and urinary tract contaminations, greater pee and hypotension.

Insulin treatment.
A few individuals who have type 2 diabetes need insulin treatment too. Previously, insulin treatment was utilized if all else fails, however today it's frequently endorsed sooner because of its advantages.

Because ordinary absorption meddles with insulin taken by mouth, insulin must be infused. Contingent upon your necessities, your specialist might endorse a blend of insulin types to use for the duration of the day and night. Regularly, individuals with type 2 diabetes begin insulin use with one long-acting shot during the evening. Insulin infusions include utilizing a fine needle and syringe or an insulin pen injector a gadget that seems to be like an ink pen, aside from the cartridge is loaded with insulin.

There are numerous types of insulin, and they every work differently. Choices include:

Insulin glulisine (Apidra)

Insulin lispro (Humalog)

Insulin aspart (Novolog)

Insulin glargine (Lantus)

Insulin detemir (Levemir)

Insulin isophane (Humulin N, Novolin N)

Talk about the advantages and disadvantages of various medications with your specialist. Together you can choose which drug is best for you subsequent to considering numerous elements, including costs and different parts of your wellbeing. Notwithstanding diabetes drugs, your specialist may endorse low-measurements headache medicine treatment and also circulatory strain and cholesterol-bringing solutions down to counteract heart and vein malady.

Bariatric surgery

If that you have type 2 diabetes and your body mass list (BMI) is more prominent than 35, you might be a possibility for weight reduction surgery (bariatric surgery). Glucose levels come back to ordinary in 55 to 95 percent of individuals with diabetes, contingent upon the strategy performed. Surgeries that sidestep a bit of the small digestive tract have a greater amount of an impact on glucose levels than do other weight reduction surgeries.

Disadvantages to the surgery incorporate its high cost, and there are dangers included, including a danger of death. Moreover, uncommon way of life changes are required and long haul difficulties might incorporate nourishing inadequacies and osteoporosis.

Ladies with type 2 diabetes might need to modify their treatment during pregnancy. Numerous ladies will require insulin treatment during pregnancy. Cholesterol-bringing down pharmaceuticals and some circulatory strain drugs can't be utilized during pregnancy. If that you have indications of diabetic retinopathy, it might compound during pregnancy. Visit your ophthalmologist during the first trimester of your pregnancy and at one year baby blues.

Indications of inconvenience

Because such a variety of variables can influence your glucose, issues once in a while emerge that require quick care, for example,

High glucose (hyperglycemia).
Your glucose level can ascend for some reasons, including eating excessively, being wiped out or not sufficiently taking glucose-bringing down solution. Check your glucose level regularly, and look for signs and indications of high glucose — successive pee, greater thirst, dry mouth, obscured vision, exhaustion and sickness. If that you have hyperglycemia, you'll have to modify your dinner arrangement, drugs or both.

Hyperglycemic hyperosmolar nonketotic disorder (HHNS).
Signs and side effects of this life-undermining condition incorporate a glucose perusing higher than 600 mg/dL (33.3 mmol/L), dry mouth, amazing thirst, fever more prominent than 101 F (38 C), laziness, disarray, vision misfortune, mind flights and dull pee. Your glucose screen will be unable to give you a precise perusing at such abnormal states and might rather simply read "high."

HHNS is caused by high as can be glucose that turns blood thick and syrupy. It has a tendency to be more normal in more established individuals with type 2 diabetes, and it's frequently went before by a disease or contamination. HHNS for the most part creates over days or weeks. Call your specialist or look for prompt therapeutic consideration if that you have signs or side effects of this condition.

Greater ketones in your pee (diabetic ketoacidosis). If that your cells are famished for vitality, your body might start to separate fat. This produces dangerous acids known as ketones. Look for thirst or an extremely dry mouth, incessant pee, regurgitating, shortness of breath, weakness and fruity-noticing breath. You can check your pee for overabundance ketones with an over-the-counter ketones test unit. If that you have overabundance ketones in your pee, counsel your specialist immediately or look for crisis care. This condition is more normal in individuals with type 1 diabetes yet can in some cases happen in individuals with type 2 diabetes.

Low glucose (hypoglycemia).
If that your glucose level drops underneath your objective range, it's known as low glucose (hypoglycemia). Your glucose level can drop for some reasons, including skirting a feast, unintentionally taking more solution than expected or getting more physical action than ordinary. Low glucose is in all probability if that you take glucose-bringing down medicines that advance the discharge of insulin or in case you're taking insulin.

Check your glucose level routinely, and look for signs and manifestations of low glucose — sweating, instability, shortcoming, hunger, wooziness, migraine, obscured vision, heart palpitations, slurred discourse, laziness, perplexity and seizures.

If that you create hypoglycemia during the night, you may wake with sweat-splashed nightgown or a migraine. Because of a characteristic bounce back impact, evening hypoglycemia may cause a surprisingly high glucose perusing first thing in the morning.

If that you have signs or side effects of low glucose, drink or eat something that will rapidly raise your glucose level — organic product juice, glucose tablets, hard sweet, standard (not eat less) pop or another wellspring of sugar. Retest in 15 minutes to make certain your blood glucose levels have standardized.

If that they haven't, treat again and retest in an additional 15 minutes. If that you lose cognizance, a relative or close contact might need to give you a crisis infusion of glucagon, a hormone that empowers the arrival of sugar into the blood.

Elective prescription

Various option prescription substances have been appeared to enhance insulin affectability in a few studies, while different studies neglect to discover any advantage for glucose control or in bringing down A1C levels. Because of the clashing discoveries, no option treatments are prescribed to help with glucose administration.

If that you choose to attempt an option treatment, don't quit taking the medicines that your specialist has endorsed. Make certain to examine the utilization of any of these treatments with your specialist to ensure that they won't cause unfriendly responses or associate with your medicines.

No medicines — elective or ordinary — can cure diabetes. So it's important that individuals who are utilizing insulin treatment for diabetes don't quit utilizing insulin unless coordinated to do as such by their physicians.

Rolling out way of life improvements

In case you're determined to have type 2 diabetes, you'll have to take care of your wellbeing painstakingly for whatever is left of your life.

This might appear to be overwhelming, however your diabetes care group will have the capacity to give you bolster and counsel about all parts of your treatment.

In the wake of being determined to have type 2 diabetes, or in case you're at danger of building up the condition, the initial step is to take a gander at your eating routine and way of life, and roll out any essential improvements.

Three noteworthy regions that you'll have to take a gander at are your:

By eating strongly, getting in shape (in case you're overweight) and practicing consistently you might have the capacity to keep your blood glucose at a sheltered and sound level without the requirement for different types of treatment.

Diet

Expanding the measure of fiber in your eating routine and diminishing your fat admission, especially soaked fat, can counteract type 2 diabetes, and additionally deal with the condition if that you as of now have it. You ought to:

Increase your utilization of high-fiber sustenances, for example, wholegrain bread and oats, beans and lentils, and foods grown from the ground pick nourishments that are low in fat – supplant margarine, ghee and coconut oil with low-fat spreads and vegetable oil

pick skimmed and semi-skimmed drain, and low-fat yoghurts

eat angle and incline meat as opposed to greasy or handled meat, for example, hotdogs and burgers

barbecue, prepare, poach or steam sustenance as opposed to broiling or cooking it

stay away from high-fat sustenances, for example, mayonnaise, chips, crisps, pasties, poppadums and samosas

eat organic product, unsalted nuts and low-fat yoghurts as snacks rather than cakes, rolls, bombay blend or crisps

The Diabetes UK site has more data and counsel about adhering to a good diet.

Weight

In case you're overweight or large (you have a body mass record (BMI) of 30 or over), you ought to shed pounds, by step by step by lessening your calorie allow and turning out to be all the more physically dynamic (see underneath).

Losing 5-10% of your general body weight through the span of a year is a practical starting target. You ought to plan to keep on getting thinner until you've accomplished and kept up a BMI inside of the sound reach, which is:

18.5-24.9kg/m² for the all inclusive community

18.5-22.9kg/m² for individuals of south Asian or Chinese inception ('south Asian' implies Bangladesh, Bhutan, India, Indian-Caribbean, Maldives, Nepal, Pakistan and Sri Lanka)

If that you have a BMI of 30kg/m² or more (27.5kg/m² or more for individuals of south Asian or Chinese starting point), you require an organized health improvement plan, which ought to shape part of a serious way of life change program.

To offer you some assistance with achieving changes in your conduct, you might be alluded to a dietitician or a comparative human services proficient for an individual appraisal and customized guidance about eating routine and physical action.

Physical action

Being physically dynamic is critical in averting or overseeing type 2 diabetes. For grown-ups who are 19-64 years old, the administration prescribes at least:

150 minutes (2 hours and 30 minutes) of "moderate-power" high-impact movement –, for example, cycling or quick strolling – a week, which can be taken in sessions of 10 minutes or more, and muscle-reinforcing exercises on two or more days a week that work all

significant muscle bunches (legs, hips, back, tummy (mid-region), mid-section, bears and arms)

An option proposal is to do at least: 75 minutes of "incredible power" vigorous movement, for example, running or a session of tennis consistently, and muscle-fortifying exercises on two or more days a week that work all significant muscle bunches (legs, hips, back, belly, mid-section, bears and arms)

In situations where the above movement levels are unlikely, even little increments in physical action will be valuable to your wellbeing and go about as a premise for future enhancements.

Diminish the measure of time spent staring at the TV or sitting before a PC. Going for a day by day walk – for instance, during your meal break – is a decent method for bringing normal physical action into your calendar. In case you're overweight or stout (see above), you might should be all the more physically dynamic to offer you some assistance with losing weight and keep up weight reduction.

Your GP, diabetes care group or dietician can give you more data and exhortation about shedding pounds and turning out to be all the more physically dynamic.

The Diabetes UK site has more data and guidance about getting dynamic and staying dynamic.

Medications for type 2 diabetes

stow away

Type 2 diabetes normally deteriorates after some time. Rolling out way of life improvements, for example, conforming your eating routine and taking more work out, might offer you some assistance with controlling your blood glucose levels at to begin with, yet they not be sufficient in the long haul.

You might in the end need to take prescription to control your blood glucose levels. At first, this will as a rule be as tablets, and can now and again be a mix of more than one type of tablet. It might likewise incorporate insulin or other pharmaceutical that you infuse.

Metformin

Metformin is normally the first drug that is utilized to treat type 2 diabetes. It works by decreasing the measure of glucose that your liver discharges into your circulation system. It additionally makes your body's cells more receptive to insulin.

Metformin is suggested for grown-ups with a high danger of creating type 2 diabetes, whose blood glucose is as yet advancing towards type 2 diabetes, in spite of rolling out fundamental way of life improvements.

In case you're overweight, it's additionally likely you'll recommended metformin. Not at all like some different solutions used to treat type 2 diabetes, metformin shouldn't cause extra weight pick up.

Nonetheless, it can some of the time cause gentle reactions, for example, queasiness and loose bowels, and you will most likely be unable to take it if that you have kidney harm.

Sulphonylureas

Sulphonylureas build the measure of insulin that is created by your pancreas. Cases of sulphonylureas include:

glibenclduringe

gliclazide

glimepiride

glipizide

gliquidone

You might be recommended one of these meds if that you can't take metformin, or if that you aren't overweight. On the other hand, you might be endorsed sulphonylurea and metformin if metformin doesn't control blood glucose all alone.

Sulphonylureas can expand the danger of hypoglycaemia (low glucose), because they build the measure of insulin in your body. They can likewise in some cases cause reactions including weight pick up, queasiness and looseness of the bowels.

Glitazones (thiazolidinediones, TZDs)

Thiazolidinedione medications (pioglitazone) make your body's cells more delicate to insulin so that more glucose is taken from your blood.

They're typically utilized as a part of blend with metformin or sulphonylureas, or both. They might cause weight pick up and lower leg swelling (oedema). You shouldn't take pioglitazone if that you have heart disappointment or a high danger of bone crack.

Another thiazolidinedione, rosiglitazone, was pulled back from use in 2010 because of an greater danger of cardiovascular issue, including heart assault and heart disappointment.

Gliptins (DPP-4 inhibitors)

Gliptins work by keeping the breakdown of a normally happening hormone called GLP-1. GLP-1 offers the body some assistance with producing insulin in light of high blood glucose levels, yet is quickly separated.

By keeping this breakdown, the gliptins (linagliptin, saxagliptin, sitagliptin and vildagliptin) anticipate high blood glucose levels, however don't bring about scenes of hypoglycaemia.

You might be recommended a gliptin in case you can't take sulphonylureas or glitazones, or in blend with them. They're not connected with weight pick up.

GLP-1 agonists

Exenatide is a GLP-1 agonist, an injectable treatment that demonstrations similarly to the characteristic hormone GLP-1 (see the area on gliptins, above). It's infused twice per day and supports insulin creation when there are high blood glucose levels, lessening blood glucose without the danger of hypoglycaemia scenes ("hypos"). It additionally prompts small weight reduction in numerous individuals who take it. It's basically utilized as a part of individuals on metformin in addition to sulphonylurea, who are large. An once-week by week item has likewise been presented.

Another GLP-1 agonist called liraglutide is an once-day by day infusion (exenatide is given twice every day). Like exenatide, liraglutide is primarily utilized for individuals on metformin in addition to sulphonylurea, who are corpulent, and in clinical trials it's been appeared to cause small weight reduction.

Acarbose

Acarbose keeps your blood glucose level from expanding a lot after you eat a dinner. It backs off the rate at which your digestive framework separates starches into glucose. Acarbose isn't regularly used to treat type 2 diabetes because it ordinarily causes symptoms, for example, bloating and the runs. Nonetheless, it might be recommended if that you can't take different types of prescription for type 2 diabetes.

Nateglinide and repaglinide

Nateglinide and repaglinide empower the arrival of insulin by your pancreas. They're not ordinarily utilized, but rather might be a choice if that you have suppers at sporadic times. This is because their belongings don't keep going long, yet they're successful when taken just before you eat.

Nateglinide and repaglinide can cause symptoms, for example, weight pick up and hypoglycaemia .

Chapter 6

Natural cure for diabetes
Diabetes treatment can incorporate numerous components, including conventional prescriptions, alternative pharmaceutical, and common cures.

Alternative treatments envelop an type of controls that incorporate everything from eating regimen and activity to mental molding and way of life changes. Illustrations of option medications incorporate needle therapy, guided symbolism, chiropractic medicines, yoga, entrancing, biofeedback, fragrance based treatment, unwinding works out, home grown cures, back rub, and numerous others.

The National Center for Complementary and Alternative Medicine, part of the National Institutes of Health, characterizes reciprocal and option medication as a "gathering of differing therapeutic and human services frameworks, practices, and items that are not without further ado thought to be a piece of customary solution." Complementary pharmaceutical is utilized with ordinary medicines, while alternative prescription is utilized rather than traditional drug.

A few individuals with diabetes use corresponding or alternative treatments to treat diabetes. Albeit some of these treatments might be powerful, others can be incapable or even hurtful. Patients who use correlative and option pharmaceutical need to tell their human services suppliers what they are doing.

Acupunture

Acupunture
is a system in which a professional embeds slight needles into assigned focuses on the skin. A few researchers say that needle therapy triggers the arrival of the body's common painkillers. Needle therapy has been appeared to offer help from perpetual agony. Needle therapy is here and there utilized by individuals with neuropathy, the agonizing nerve harm of diabetes.

Biofeedback

Biofeedback is a strategy that offers a man some assistance with becoming more mindful of and figure out how to manage the body's reaction to torment. This option treatment underlines unwinding and push decrease procedures.

Guided symbolism is an unwinding method that a few experts who use biofeedback likewise rehearse. With guided symbolism, a man considers serene mental pictures, for example, sea waves. A man might likewise incorporate the pictures of controlling or curing an incessant infection, for example, diabetes. Individuals utilizing this method say these positive pictures can facilitate their condition.

What Natural Dietary Supplements Are Used for Diabetes Treatment?

Chromium

The advantage of included chromium for diabetes has been considered and wrangled for quite a while. A few studies report that chromium supplements might enhance diabetes control. Chromium is expected to make glucose resistance variable, which offers insulin some assistance with improving its activity. Because of deficient data on the utilization of chromium to treat diabetes, no suggestions for supplementation exist.

Ginseng

A few types of plants are alluded to as ginseng, however most investigations of ginseng and diabetes have utilized American ginseng. Those studies have demonstrated some sugar-bringing down impacts in fasting and after-dinner glucose levels and also in A1c levels (normal glucose levels over a three-month period). On the other hand, bigger and all the more long haul studies are required before general suggestions for utilization of ginseng can be made. Scientists additionally have discovered that the measure of sugar-bringing down compound in ginseng plants changes generally.

Magnesium

Despite the fact that the relationship in the middle of magnesium and diabetes has been concentrated on for quite a long time, it is not yet completely caught on. Contemplates demonstrate that an insufficiency in magnesium might intensify glucose control in type 2 diabetes. Researchers say that an insufficiency of magnesium interferes with insulin emission in the pancreas and expands insulin resistance in the body's tissues. Proof recommends that a lack of magnesium might add to specific diabetes inconveniences. A late investigation demonstrated that individuals with higher dietary admissions of magnesium (through utilization of entire grains, nuts, and green verdant vegetables) had a diminished danger of type 2 diabetes.

Vanadium

Vanadium is a compound found in small sums in plants and creatures. Early studies demonstrated that vanadium standardized glucose levels in creatures with type 1 and type 2 diabetes. A late study found that when individuals with diabetes were given vanadium, they added to an unobtrusive increment in insulin affectability and could diminish their insulin necessities. As of now scientists need to see how vanadium functions in the body, find potential reactions, and build up safe measurements.

Coenzyme Q10

Coenzyme Q10, frequently alluded to as CoQ10 (different names incorporate ubiquinone and ubiquinol) is a vitamin-like substance. CoQ10 offers cells some assistance with making vitality and goes about as a cancer prevention agent. Meats and fish contain little measures of CoQ10. Supplements are advertised as tablets and cases. The confirmation is not adequate to assess CoQ10's viability as an integral or option treatment for diabetes. CoQ10 has not been appeared to influence glucose control.

What Plant Foods Are Used for Diabetes Treatment?

The accompanying plant nourishments are now and again utilized for diabetes treatment, especially for those with type 2 diabetes.

Brewer's yeast

Buckwheat

Broccoli and other related greens

Cinnamon

Cloves

Espresso

Okra

Peas

Fenugreek seeds

Sage

Most plant sustenances are rich in fiber, vitamins, and minerals, which are vital to great wellbeing in individuals with diabetes. Some uncovering new studies demonstrate that specific plant nourishments - cinnamon, cloves, and espresso - might really help in battling aggravation and help insulin, the hormone that aides controls glucose. Thinks about have demonstrated that cinnamon concentrates can enhance sugar digestion system, activating insulin discharge, which additionally influences cholesterolmetabolism. Clove oil removes (eugenol) have been found to enhance the capacity of insulin and to lower glucose, all out cholesterol, LDL, and triglycerides. Late discoveries show that an obscure compound in espresso (not caffeine) might improve insulin affectability and lessen the danger of creating type 2 diabetes.

Still, the logical proof so far does not bolster the part of garlic, ginger, ginseng, hawthorn, or weed in profiting glucose control in individuals with diabetes. If that you have diabetes and are considering taking any of these home grown substances for diabetes treatment, make certain you converse with your specialist before you take them.

What Weight Control Substances Are Used for Diabetes Treatment?

The accompanying plant nourishments are some of the time utilized for diabetes treatment, especially for those with type 2 diabetes.

Flavors and Herbs to Pump Up the Flavor

Since weight and diabetes are connected, numerous individuals with diabetes swing to common option treatments for diabetes treatment, especially those that claim to help with weight reduction, including:

Chitosan

Garcinia cambogia (hydroxycitric corrosive)

Chromium

Pyruvate

Germander

Momordica charantia

Sauropus androgynus

Aristolochic corrosive

What's more, transdermal (skin patch) frameworks and also oral showers have been produced to purportedly lessen hankering and encourage weight reduction. One patch framework utilizes homeopathic measures of 29 unique mixes to decrease craving. What is all that really matters? There's not one distributed study accessible on its viability.

Are Herbs Really Safe for Diabetes Treatment?

In 2003, ephedrine - otherwise called mama huang - turned into the first home grown stimulant ever banned by the FDA. A famous segment of over-the-stabilizer misfortune drugs, ephedrine was found to have a few advantages. Be that as it may, the confirmation of its capacity to cause damage was significantly all the more convincing. In high dosages, ephedrine has been known not sleep deprivation (trouble falling and staying unconscious), hypertension, glaucoma, and urinary maintenance. This home grown supplement has additionally been connected with various instances of stroke.

Chitosan is gotten from seashells and can tie to fat and keep its assimilation. In spite of the fact that it is said to encourage weight reduction, accessible concentrates hitherto have not been empowering.

Germander, Momordica charantia, Sauropus androgynus, and aristolochic corrosive have been connected with liver sickness, pneumonic malady, and kidney ailment.

The other alleged "weight cures" recorded have not been thoroughly considered, and those that been checked on have yielded baffling results.

Additionally, a late study of home grown arrangements for heftiness found that numerous arrangements contained lead or arsenic and other dangerous metals. Some additionally contain other undeclared fixings. Every so often, there was mixed up plant way of life also.

What to Consider Before Using Natural Therapies for Diabetes Treatment

Before you consider utilizing a characteristic treatment for diabetes treatment, make sure to consider the accompanying:

Talk about any medications you utilize, including natural items, with your specialist before taking them.

If that you encounter symptoms, for example, queasiness, retching, fast pulse, uneasiness, a sleeping disorder, looseness of the bowels, or skin rashes, quit taking the natural item and tell your specialist quickly.

Stay away from arrangements made with more than one herb.

.

Chapter 7

Food and nutrition

Diabetes is on the ascent, yet most cases are preventable with sound way of life changes. Some can even be turned around. Finding a way to avert and control diabetes doesn't mean living in hardship; it implies eating a wonderful, adjusted eating routine that will likewise help your vitality and enhance your state of mind. You don't need to surrender desserts completely or leave yourself to a lifetime of dull food. With these tips, you can in any case take delight from your dinners without feeling ravenous or denied.

Taking control of diabetes

Whether you're attempting to avoid or control diabetes, there is some uplifting news. You can have a major effect with solid way of life changes. The most imperative thing you can accomplish for your wellbeing is to get more fit—yet you don't need to lose all your additional pounds to begin profiting. Specialists say that losing only 5% to 10% of your aggregate weight can offer you bring down your blood some assistance with sugaring impressively, and also bring down your circulatory strain and cholesterol levels. Getting more fit and eating more advantageous can likewise profoundly affect your state of mind, vitality levels, and feeling of wellbeing.

It's not very late to roll out a positive improvement, regardless of the possibility that you've effectively created diabetes. The primary concern is that you have more control over your wellbeing than you might suspect.

The significance of getting in shape in the "right" places

The greatest danger variable for creating diabetes is being overweight, however not all muscle to fat quotients is made equivalent. Your danger is higher if that you tend to bear your weight your mid-region— the alleged "extra tire"— instead of your hips and thighs. So why are "apple" formed individuals more at danger than "pears"?

"Pears" store the majority of their fat close beneath the skin. "Apples" store their weight around their center, quite a bit of it profound inside of the paunch encompassing their stomach organs and liver. This type of profound fat is firmly connected to insulin resistance and diabetes.

Truth be told, numerous studies demonstrate that waist size is a superior indicator of diabetes danger than BMI (body mass record).

You are at an greater danger of creating diabetes if that you are:

A lady with a waist boundary of 35 inches or more

A man with a waist boundary of 40 inches or more

To gauge your waist boundary, put a measuring tape around your uncovered midriff simply over your hip bone. Make certain that the tape is cozy (yet does not pack your skin) and that it is parallel to the floor. Unwind, breathe out, and measure your waist.

The risks of "sugar tummy"

Calories acquired from fructose (found in sugary refreshments, for example, pop, vitality and sports drinks, espresso drinks, and prepared foods like doughnuts, biscuits, oat, sweet and granola bars) will probably transform you into an "apple" by including weight around your mid-region. Curtailing sugary foods can mean a slimmer waistline and in addition a lower danger of diabetes.

What you have to think about diabetes and diet

Eating right is basic in case you're attempting to counteract or control diabetes. While activity is additionally vital, what you eat has the greatest effect with regards to weight reduction. In any case, what does eating a good fit for diabetes mean? You might be astonished to hear that your nutritional needs are for all intents and purposes the same other people: no extraordinary foods or entangled eating methodologies are fundamental.

A diabetes eating routine is just an adhering to a good diet arrange for that is high in supplements, low in fat and included sugar, and direct in calories. It is a solid eating routine for anybody! The main distinction is that you have to give careful consideration to some of your food decisions—most eminently the sugars you eat.

Myths and realities about diabetes and diet

MYTH: You should avoid sugar no matter what.

Reality: The uplifting news is that you can make the most of your most loved regards the length of you plan legitimately and limit those shrouded sugars in numerous bundled foods. Pastry doesn't need to be forbidden, insofar as it's a part of a sound feast arrange or consolidated with activity.

MYTH: A high-protein eating regimen is best.

Reality: Studies have demonstrated that eating an excess of protein, particularly creature protein, might really bring about insulin resistance, a key component in diabetes. A solid eating routine incorporates protein, sugars, and fats. Our bodies require every one of the three to work appropriately. The key is an adjusted eating routine.

MYTH: You need to cut your intake down on carbs.

Reality: Again, the key is to eat an adjusted eating routine. The serving size and the type of sugars you eat are particularly vital. Concentrate on entire grain carbs since they are a decent wellspring of fiber and they are processed gradually, keeping glucose levels all the more even.

MYTH: You'll never again have the capacity to eat regularly. You require exceptional diabetic dinners.

Reality: The standards of adhering to a good diet are the same— regardless of whether you're attempting to anticipate or control diabetes. Costly diabetic foods for the most part offer no unique advantage. You can without much of a stretch eat with your family and companions if that you eat with some restraint.

Diabetes and diet tip 1: **Choose high-fiber, moderate discharge carbs**

Starches bigly affect your glucose levels—more so than fats and proteins—yet you don't need to stay away from them. You simply should be shrewd about what types of carbs you eat.

When all is said in done, it's best to restrict profoundly refined sugars like white bread, pasta, and rice, and in addition pop, sweet, bundled dinners, and nibble foods. Center rather on high-fiber complex sugars—otherwise called moderate discharge carbs. Moderate discharge carbs keep glucose levels even on the grounds that they are processed all the more gradually, in this way keeping your body from delivering an excessive amount of insulin. They likewise give enduring vitality and offer you some assistance with staying full more.

Picking carbs that are stuffed with fiber (and don't spike your glucose)

Rather than...   Try these high-fiber choices...

White rice

Chestnut rice or wild rice

White potatoes (counting fries and pureed potatoes)

Sweet potatoes, yams, winter squash, cauliflower crush

Customary pasta

Entire wheat pasta

White bread

Entire wheat or entire grain bread

Sugary breakfast oat

High-fiber, low-sugar breakfast oat

Instant cereal

Steel-cut oats or moved oats

Cornflakes

Low-sugar wheat drops

Corn

Peas or verdant greens

Diabetes and glycemic file

The glycemic file (GI) and glycemic load offer data about how diverse foods influence glucose and insulin levels. High GI foods spike your glucose quickly, while low GI foods have minimal impact on glucose. While the GI has long been elevated as an instrument to individuals with diabetes oversee glucose and enhance their eating regimens, there are some outstanding downsides. Firstly, in spite of a lot of examination, the genuine medical advantages of utilizing the GI stay misty. Referring to glycemic file tables can make eating pointlessly confounded. At long last, the GI is not a measure of a food's empowerment. Late research recommends that by basically taking after the rules of the Mediterranean or other heart-sound weight control plans, you'll bring down your glycemic load as well as enhance the nature of your eating regimen too.

Investigate the master plan: your general eating examples are more vital than fixating on individual foods. To put it plainly, eat a greater amount of the well done and less of the terrible.

Controlling weight with the glycemic file

Specialists trust that the way to weight control lies in decreasing the measure of refined starches ("white" or "fire" foods) in your eating routine. Rather, concentrate on low GI or "coal" foods which keep you feeling more full any longer. Low-glycemic foods take more time to process so sugar is ingested all the more gradually into the circulatory system. Accordingly you're less inclined to encounter a spike in your glucose level, you'll remain satisfied for more, and are less inclined to gorge.

Maintain a strategic distance from handled foods such as prepared merchandise, sugary sweets, and bundled oat and pick rather for steel cut oats, beans, without fat low-sugar yogurt, dull green verdant vegetables, and entire grains.

Eat entire crisp natural product rather than organic product juice—pressing organic product discharges more sugar so an entire orange has a lower GI than a glass of juice.

Eat More nutritious food

Solid fats from crude nuts, olive oil, fish oils, flax seeds, entire milk dairy, or avocados

Foods grown from the ground—in a perfect world new, the more brilliant the better; entire organic product as opposed to squeezes

High-fiber oats and breads produced using entire grains or vegetables

Fish and shellfish, natural, unfenced chicken or turkey

Top notch protein, for example, eggs, beans, milk, cheddar, and unsweetened yogurt

Eat Less

Trans fats from in part hydrogenated or southern style foods; immersed fats from garbage food or handled meat

Bundled and quick foods, particularly those high in sugar and sodium, prepared merchandise, desserts, chips, treats

White bread, sugary grains, refined pastas or rice

Handled meat and red meat from creatures bolstered with anti-infection agents, development hormones, and GMO encourage

Low-fat items that have supplanted fat with included sugar, for example, without fat yogurt

Diabetes and diet tip 2: Be brilliant about desserts

Eating a diabetes-accommodating eating routine doesn't mean killing sugar inside and out, however like most grown-ups in the west, odds are you devour more sugar than is solid. If that you have diabetes, you can in any case appreciate a little serving of your most loved sweet from time to time. The key is control.

The most effective method to incorporate desserts in a diabetes-accommodating eating routine.

If that you have a sweet tooth, the considered decreasing desserts might sound nearly as awful as removing them by and large. The uplifting news is that longings do leave and inclinations change. By gradually lessening the sugar in your eating routine a little at once, you'll give your taste buds time to change and you'll have the capacity to wean yourself off the desire for desserts. Furthermore, as your dietary patterns get to be more advantageous, the sweet foods that you used to love might appear to be excessively rich or too sweet, and you'll end up desiring more beneficial alternatives.

Hold the bread (or rice or pasta) if that you need dessert. Eating desserts at a supper includes additional starches. Due to this it is best to curtail the other carb-containing foods at the same supper.

Add some solid fat to your sweet. It might appear to be outlandish to ignore the low-fat or without fat treats for their higher-fat partners. Yet, fat backs off the digestive procedure, which means glucose levels don't spike as fast. That doesn't mean, nonetheless, that you ought to go after the doughnuts. Think solid fats, for example, nutty spread, ricotta cheddar, yogurt, or a few nuts. Eat desserts with a feast, as opposed to as a stand-alone nibble. At the point when eaten all alone, desserts and treats cause your glucose to spike. Be that as it may, if that you eat them alongside other sound foods as a feature of your feast, your glucose won't ascend as quickly.

When you eat dessert, genuinely appreciate every nibble. How often have you thoughtlessly eaten your way through a pack of treats or a gigantic bit of cake? Will you truly say that you delighted in every chomp? Make the most of your liberality by eating gradually and paying consideration on the flavors and surfaces. You'll appreciate it more, in addition to you're more averse to gorge.

Traps for controling sugar

Continue with alert with regards to liquor

It's anything but difficult to think little of the measure of calories and carbs in mixed beverages, including lager and wine. What's more, mixed drinks blended with pop and squeeze can be stacked with sugar. In case you're going to drink, do as such with some restraint (close to 1 drink for every day for ladies; 2 for men), pick without calorie drink blenders, and drink just with food. In case you're diabetic, dependably screen your blood glucose, as liquor can meddle with diabetes prescription and insulin.

Decrease how much sodas, pop and squeeze you drink. A late study found that for every 12 oz. serving of a sugar-sweetened refreshment you drink a day, your danger for diabetes increments by around 15 percent. If that you miss your carbonation kick, take a stab at shimmering water with a bit of lemon or lime or a sprinkle of organic product juice. Decrease the measure of flavors and sweeteners you add to tea and espresso drinks.

Try not to supplant soaked fat with sugar. A large portion of us commit the error of supplanting sound wellsprings of immersed fat, for example, entire milk dairy, with refined carbs or sugary foods, supposing we're settling on a more advantageous decision. Low-fat doesn't as a matter of course mean solid, particularly when the fat has been supplanted by added sugar to compensate for loss of taste.

Sweeten foods yourself. Purchase unsweetened frosted tea, plain yogurt, or unflavored oats, for instance, and include sweetener (or organic product) yourself. You're prone to include far less sugar than the producer would have.

Check names and decide on low sugar items and utilize new or solidified fixings rather than canned merchandise. Be particularly mindful of the sugar substance of grains and sugary beverages.

Maintain a strategic distance from handled or bundled foods like canned soups, solidified suppers, or low-fat dinners that frequently contain shrouded sugar. Get ready more dinners at home.

While purchasing foods, for example, syrups, jams, and sauces, select items named "diminished sugar" or "no included sugar."

Decrease the measure of sugar in formulas by ¼ to ⅓. If that a formula calls for some sugar, for instance, use ⅔ or ¾ glass. You can likewise support sweetness with mint, cinnamon, nutmeg, or vanilla concentrate rather than sugar.

Find sound approaches to fulfill your sweet tooth. Rather than dessert, mix up solidified bananas for a rich, solidified treat. On the other hand appreciate a little piece of dull chocolate, as opposed to your standard milk chocolate bar.

Begin with half of the sweet you ordinarily eat, and supplant the other half with organic product.

Being brilliant about desserts is just part of the fight, however. Sugar is additionally covered up in numerous bundled foods, fast food suppers, and market staples, for example, bread, grains, sweet beverages, canned soups and vegetables, pasta sauce, margarine, instant pureed potatoes, solidified suppers, low-fat dinners, and ketchup. By decreasing the measure of shrouded sugar you expend in these types of foods can even permit you to eat a greater amount of the sweet treats you hunger for. The initial step is to figure out how to recognize shrouded sugars on food names.

Do some analyst work

Spotting included sugar food marks can require some sleuthing. Producers are required to give the aggregate sum of sugar in a serving yet don't need to delineate the amount of this sugar has been included and what amount is normally in the food. Included sugars must be incorporated the fixings list, which is exhibited in plunging request by weight. The trap is decoding which fixings are included sugars. They arrive in an assortment of pretenses. Beside the undeniable ones— sugar, nectar, molasses—included sugar can show up as agave nectar, stick gems, corn sweetener, crystalline fructose, dextrose, dissipated stick juice, fructose, high-fructose corn syrup, upset sugar, lactose, maltose, malt syrup, and the sky is the limit from there.

An astute methodology is to stay away from items that have any of these included sugars at or close to the highest priority on the rundown of fixings—or ones that have a few distinct types of sugar scattered all through the rundown. If that an item is crammed with sugar, you would hope to see "sugar" recorded in the first place, or perhaps second. In any case, food creators can fudge the rundown by including sweeteners that aren't actually called sugar. The trap is that every sweetener is recorded independently. The commitment of each included sugar might be sufficiently little that it appears fourth, fifth, or significantly facilitate down the rundown. Be that as it may, include them up and you can get an amazing measurement of included sugar.

How about we take as a case a well known oat-based oat with almonds whose bundle gloats that it is "extraordinary tasting," "heart sound" and "entire grain ensured." Here's the rundown of fixings:

Entire grain oats, entire grain wheat, chestnut sugar, almond pieces, sugar, fresh oats,* corn syrup, grain malt extricate, potassium citrate, toasted oats,* salt, malt syrup, wheat bits,* nectar, and cinnamon.

*contain sugar, high-fructose corn syrup, nectar, and/or cocoa sugar molasses.

Join cocoa sugar, sugar, corn syrup, grain malt remove, high-fructose corn syrup, nectar, chestnut sugar molasses, and malt syrup, and they mean a strong dosage of unfilled calories—more than one-quarter (27%) of this oat is included sugar, which you won't not figure from examining the fixing list. This type of figuring can be particularly dubious in breakfast grains, where the greater part of the sugars are included.

Adjusted with authorization from Reducing Sugar and Salt, a unique wellbeing report distributed by Harvard Health Publications.

Diabetes and your eating routine tip 3: Choose fats carefully

Fats can be either useful or hurtful in your eating regimen. Individuals with diabetes are at higher danger for coronary illness, so it is much more vital to be savvy about fats. A few fats are unfortunate and others have huge medical advantages. However, all fats are high in calories, so you ought to dependably watch your bit sizes.

Horrible fats – The most harming fats are trans fats, likewise called somewhat hydrogenated oils, which are made by adding hydrogen to fluid vegetable oils to make them more strong and less inclined to ruin—which is useful for food producers, and awful for you. Stay away from financially heated products, bundled nibble foods, browned food, and anything with "somewhat hydrogenated" oil in the fixings, regardless of the possibility that it cases to be trans sans fat.

Sound fats – The most secure fats are unsaturated fats, which originate from plant and angle sources, for example, olive oil, nuts, and avocados. Likewise concentrate on omega-3 unsaturated fats, which battle irritation and support cerebrum and heart wellbeing. Great sources incorporate salmon, fish, and flaxseeds.

Immersed fats – Not all soaked fat is the same. The immersed fat in entire milk dairy, coconut oil, or salmon is distinctive to the unfortunate soaked fat found in pizza, French fries, and handled meat items, which have been connected to coronary infection and tumor. Late proof proposes that expending entire fat dairy can have gainful impacts, including controlling weight.

Approaches to diminish horrible fats and include solid fats:

Rather than chips or saltines, have a go at nibbling on nuts or seeds. Add them to your morning grain or have somewhat modest bunch for a filling nibble. Nut spreads are additionally extremely fulfilling and loaded with solid fats.

Rather than browning, sear, prepare, or panfry.

Stay away from immersed fat from prepared meats, bundled dinners, and takeout food.

Change your eating routine with unfenced chicken, eggs, fish, and vegan wellsprings of protein.

If that you eat red meat, attempt to search for "natural" and "grass-encouraged".

Use frosty squeezed additional virgin olive oil to dress plates of mixed greens, cooked vegetables, or pasta dishes. Additionally utilize olive oil for stovetop cooking, as opposed to stick margarine or canola oil.

Dress your own serving of mixed greens. Business serving of mixed greens dressings are regularly high in calories, soaked fat, or made with harmed trans fat oils. Make your own sound dressings with additional virgin olive oil, flaxseed oil, or sesame oil.

Eat more avocados. Attempt them in sandwiches or servings of mixed greens or make guacamole. Alongside being stacked with heart and cerebrum sound fats, they make for a filling and fulfilling dinner.

Appreciate full-fat dairy and pick natural or crude milk, cheddar, margarine, and yogurt when conceivable.

Diabetes and diet tip 4: Eat frequently and keep a food journal

In case you're overweight, you might be urged to note that you just need to lose 7% of your body weight to slice your danger of diabetes down the middle. Also, you don't need to fanatically check calories or starve yourself to do it. Research demonstrates that the two most supportive systems include taking after a customary eating plan and recording what you eat.

What would it be a good idea for me to eat?

ladies picking food

Individuals with diabetes ought to take after the Australian Dietary Guidelines. Eating the prescribed measure of food from the five food gatherings will give you the supplements you should be sound and anticipate endless infections, for example, heftiness and coronary illness.

Grown-ups

Kids

To deal with your diabetes:

Eat consistent suppers and spread them equitably for the duration of the day

Eat an eating routine lower in fat, especially immersed fat

If that you take insulin or diabetes tablets, you might need between feast snacks

Recognize that everybody's needs are distinctive. All individuals with diabetes ought to see an Accredited Practicing Dietitian in conjunction with their diabetes group for individualized counsel. Perused our position explanation 'One Diet Does Not Fit All'.

Vitality equalization

Coordinating the measure of food you eat with the measure of vitality you smolder through movement and activity is vital. Putting an excessive amount of fuel in your body can prompt weight pick up. Being overweight or corpulent can make it hard to deal with your diabetes and can build the danger of coronary illness, stroke and growth.

Limit foods high in vitality, for example, take away foods, sweet scones, cakes, sugar sweetened beverages and natural product juice, lollies, chocolate and appetizing snacks. A few individuals have a sound eating routine however eat excessively. Lessening your segment size is one approach to diminish the measure of vitality you eat. Being dynamic has numerous advantages. Alongside adhering to a good diet, customary physical action can offer you to deal with your blood glucose some assistance with leveling, decrease your blood fats (cholesterol and triglycerides) and keep up a solid weight.

Fat

Fats have the most astounding vitality (kilojoule or calorie) substance of all foods. Eating an excess of fat can make you put on weight, which might make it more hard to oversee blood glucose levels. Our bodies require some fat for good wellbeing yet the type of fat you pick is imperative.

saturated fat

It is essential to constrain soaked fat since it raises your LDL ('awful') cholesterol levels. Soaked fat is found in creature foods like greasy meat, drain, spread and cheddar. Vegetable fats that are immersed incorporate palm oil (found in strong cooking fats, nibble foods or accommodation foods) and coconut items, for example, copha, coconut drain or cream.

To reduce saturated fat in your diet:

Pick diminished or low-fat milk, yogurt, cheddar, frozen yogurt and custard

Pick incline meat and trim any fat off before cooking

Expel the skin from chicken, duck and other poultry (where conceivable, before cooking)

Abstain from utilizing spread, grease, dribbling, cream, sharp cream, copha, coconut milk, coconut cream and hard cooking margarines

Limit baked goods, cakes, puddings, chocolate and cream bread rolls to exceptional events

Limit pre-bundled bread rolls, exquisite parcel snacks, cakes, solidified and accommodation dinners

Limit the utilization of prepared store meats (devon/polony/fritz/lunch get-together meat, chicken roll, salami and so on) and wieners

Maintain a strategic distance from browned takeaway foods, for example, chips, broiled chicken and battered fish and pick BBQ chicken (without the skin) and flame broiled fish

Maintain a strategic distance from pies, hotdog rolls and baked goods

As opposed to smooth sauces or dressings, pick those that depend on tomato, soy or other low fat fixings

Limit velvety style soups.

Polyunsaturated and monounsaturated fats

Eating little measures of polyunsaturated and monounsaturated fats can guarantee you get the vital unsaturated fats and vitamins your body needs.

Polyunsaturated fats include:

Polyunsaturated margarines (check the name for the word 'polyunsaturated')

Sunflower, safflower, soybean, corn, cottonseed, grapeseed and sesame oils

The fat found in slick fish, for example, herring, mackerel, sardine, salmon and fish.

Monounsaturated fats include:

Canola and olive oils

A few margarines

Avocado.
Seeds, nuts, nut spreads and shelled nut oil contain a blend of polyunsaturated and monounsaturated fat.

Thoughts for getting a charge out of solid fats

Fish-with-Lentil-Spinach-Salad

Panfry meat and vegetables in a little canola oil (or oil shower) with garlic or bean stew

Dress a serving of mixed greens or steamed vegetables with somewhat olive oil and lemon juice or vinegar

Sprinkle sesame seeds on steamed vegetables

Use linseed bread and spread a little canola margarine

Nibble on a modest bunch of unsalted nuts, or add some to a panfry or plate of mixed greens

Spread avocado on sandwiches and toast, or add to a serving of mixed greens

Eat more fish (no less than three times each week) since it contains an extraordinary type of fat (omega-3) that is useful for your heart.

Accomplish more dry cooking, flame broiling, microwaving and mix singing in a non-stick dish

Maintain a strategic distance from rotisserie, battered and crumbed foods

Sugar

Sugar foods assume a vital part in our eating regimen. They are the best vitality hotspot for your body, particularly your mind. At the point when starches are processed they separate to shape glucose in the circulation system. Insulin takes the glucose out of the blood and places it into the muscles, liver and different cells in the body where it is utilized to give vitality. Most starch containing foods are likewise great wellsprings of fiber, vitamins and minerals which keep our body and insides sound.

Of the three key supplements in our food – fat, protein and sugar, starch is the supplement that will have the greatest effect on your blood glucose levels. The impact of sugar will rely on upon i) the measure of starch you eat and ii) the type of starch you eat.

Everybody's starch needs are distinctive relying upon your sexual orientation, how dynamic you are, your age and your body weight. Anybody with diabetes ought to see an Accredited Practicing Dietitian to work out the measure of sugar to eat at every supper and nibble.

For a few individuals, a lower starch eating routine might help with diabetes administration. If that you are considering lessening the sugar substance of your eating regimen, counsel your human services group for individualized guidance.

If that you eat standard dinners and spread your sugar foods uniformly for the duration of the day, you will keep up your vitality levels without bringing on vast ascents in your blood glucose levels. If that you take insulin or diabetes tablets, you might need between dinner snacks. Talk about this with your specialist, dietitian or Credentialled Diabetes Educator.

All sugar foods are processed to deliver glucose yet they do as such at various rates – some moderate, some quick. The glycemic record or GI is a method for depicting how rapidly a starch food is processed and enters the circulatory system.

Low GI sugar foods enter the circulation system gradually and have less of an effect on blood glucose levels. Cases of low GI foods incorporate customary moved oats, thick wholegrain breads, lentils and vegetables, sweet potato, milk, yogurt, pasta and most types of crisp organic product. The type of sugar you eat is critical as some can bring about higher blood glucose in the wake of eating. The best blend is to eat moderate measures of high fiber low GI sugars.

Starch

A good dieting arrangement for diabetes can incorporate some sugar. It is alright to have a sprinkle of sugar on porridge or a scratch of jam on some low GI high fiber bread. In any case, foods that are high in included sugars and poor wellsprings of different supplements ought to be devoured sparingly. Specifically, restrain high vitality foods, for example, desserts, lollies and standard soda pops. Some sugar might likewise be utilized as a part of cooking and numerous formulas can be adjusted to utilize not exactly the sum expressed or substituted with an option sweetener. Select formulas that are low in fat (especially soaked fat) and contain some fiber.

Alternative sweeteners

As specified above little measures of sugar as a component of an adjusted supper arrangement shouldn't largy affect blood glucose levels. However sweeteners, for example, Equal, Stevia, Sugarine and Splenda can be utilized as a part of spot of sugar particularly if that they are supplanting a lot of sugar. Foods and drinks that have been sweetened with an option sweetener, for example, eat less sodas and cordials, without sugar lollies and so forth., are likewise best delighted in once in a while, as they don't have any nutritional advantage and might frequently assume the position of more nutritious foods and beverages, for example, natural products, vegetables, dairy, nuts and water.

Protein

Protein foods are required by the body for development and repair. Protein does not separate into glucose, so it doesn't straightforwardly raise blood glucose levels.

The principal protein foods are:

Meats, chicken, fish, and tofu

Eggs

Nuts and seeds

Cheddar

There are some protein foods which additionally contain starch, for example, milk, yogurt, lentils and vegetables which will affect blood glucose levels however these ought to still be incorporated as a major aspect of a sound eating regimen.

Drink water

Water is required for the greater part of the body's capacities and the body should be kept hydrated each day. Water is the best drink to have in light of the fact that it contains no additional kilojoules and won't affect your blood glucose levels. Other great decisions are:

Tea, espresso, natural tea, water, pop water, plain mineral water

If that you need a sweet drink at times items marked "eating regimen" or 'low joule'

If that you drink liquor restrain your admission to close to 2 standard beverages for every day with some liquor free days every week.

Medicinal nutrition treatment is a necessary segment of diabetes administration and of diabetes self-administration instruction. Yet numerous misguided judgments exist concerning nutrition and diabetes. In addition, in clinical practice, nutrition proposals that have practically zero supporting confirmation have been are as yet being given to persons with diabetes. In like manner, this position articulation gives proof based standards and proposals for diabetes medicinal nutrition treatment. The method of reasoning for this position explanation is talked about in the American Diabetes Association specialized audit "Proof Based Nutrition Principles and Recommendations for the Treatment and Prevention of Diabetes and Related Complications," which examines in point of interest the distributed examination for every rule and suggestion .

Verifiably, nutrition suggestions for diabetes and related difficulties depended on logical information, clinical experience, and master accord; in any case, it was frequently hard to perceive the level of confirmation used to build the proposals. To address this issue, the 2002 specialized audit and this position articulation give standards and suggestions grouped by level of confirmation accessible utilizing the American Diabetes Association proof reviewing framework. On the other hand, the best accessible proof should even now consider individual circumstances, inclinations, and social and ethnic inclinations, and the individual with diabetes ought to be included in the choice making process. The objective of proof based proposals is to enhance diabetes care by expanding the consciousness of clinicians and persons with diabetes about valuable nutrition treatments.

In light of the many-sided quality of nutrition issues, it is suggested that an enlisted dietitian, proficient and talented in executing nutrition treatment into diabetes administration and instruction, be the colleague giving medicinal nutrition treatment. On the other hand, it is fundamental that all colleagues learned about nutrition treatment and steady of the individual with diabetes who needs to roll out way of life improvements.

Objectives of therapeutic nutrition treatment that apply to all persons with diabetes are as per the following:

Blood glucose levels in the ordinary reach or as near typical as is securely conceivable to forestall or diminish the danger for difficulties of diabetes.

A lipid and lipoprotein profile that decreases the danger for macrovascular infection.

Pulse levels that decrease the danger for vascular malady.

Avoid and treat the constant confusions of diabetes. Adjust supplement admission and way of life as fitting for the counteractive action and treatment of heftiness, dyslipidemia, cardiovascular sickness, hypertension, and nephropathy.

Enhance wellbeing through sound food decisions and physical action.

Address individual nutritional needs thinking about individual and social inclinations and way of life while regarding the individual's wishes and eagerness to change.

Objectives of restorative nutrition treatment that apply to particular circumstances incorporate the accompanying:

For youth with type 1 diabetes, to give sufficient vitality to guarantee ordinary development and improvement, incorporate insulin regimens into normal eating and physical movement propensities.

For youth with type 2 diabetes, to encourage changes in eating and physical action propensities that diminish insulin resistance and enhance metabolic status.

For pregnant and lactating ladies, to give sufficient vitality and supplements required for ideal results.

For more established grown-ups, to accommodate the nutritional and psychosocial needs of a maturing person. For people treated with insulin or insulin secretagogues, to give self-administration training to treatment (and anticipation) of hypoglycemia, intense ailments, and exercise-related blood glucose issues. For people at danger for diabetes, to abatement hazard by empowering physical action and advancing food decisions that encourage moderate weight reduction or if nothing else anticipate weight pick up.

Medicinal NUTRITION THERAPY FOR TYPE 1 AND TYPE 2 DIABETES

Sugar and diabetes

At the point when alluding to basic food sugars, the accompanying terms are favored: sugars, starch, and fiber. Terms, for example, straightforward sugars, complex starches, and quick acting sugars are not very much characterized and ought to be maintained a strategic distance from. Examines in solid subjects and those at danger for type 2 diabetes bolster the significance of including foods containing sugar, especially from entire grains, natural products, vegetables, and low-fat milk in the eating routine of individuals with diabetes.

Various variables impact glycemic reactions to foods, including the measure of starch, type of sugar (glucose, fructose, sucrose, lactose), nature of the starch (amylose, amylopectin, safe starch), cooking and food handling (level of starch gelantinization, molecule size, cell structure), and food structure, and in addition other food segments (fat and regular substances that moderate absorption—lectins, phytates, tannins, and starch-protein and starch-lipid blends). Fasting and preprandial glucose focuses, the seriousness of glucose prejudice, and the second dinner or lente impact of starch are different variables influencing the glycemic reaction to foods. Then again, in persons with type 1 or type 2 diabetes, ingestion of an assortment of starches or sucrose, both intensely and for up to 6 weeks, delivered no noteworthy contrasts in glycemic reaction if the measure of sugar was comparative. Thinks about in controlled settings and examines in free-living subjects created comparative results. In this manner, the aggregate sum of starch in dinners and snacks will be more critical than the source or the type. Contemplates in subjects with type 1 diabetes demonstrate a solid relationship between the premeal insulin measurement and the postprandial reaction to the aggregate starch substance of the supper. In this manner, the premeal insulin measurements ought to be balanced for the sugar substance of the feast. For people accepting settled measurements of insulin, everyday consistency in the measure of sugar is imperative.

In persons with type 2 diabetes, on weight support diets, supplanting sugar with monounsaturated fat diminishes postprandial glycemia and triglyceridemia. On the other hand, there is worry that greater fat admission in not indispensable eating regimens might advance weight pick up. Hence, the commitments of sugar and monounsaturated fat to vitality admission ought to be individualized in view of nutrition evaluation, metabolic profiles, and treatment objectives.

Glycemic record.
Albeit low glycemic record eating methodologies might decrease postprandial glycemia, the capacity of people to keep up these eating methodologies long haul (and in this way accomplish glycemic

advantage) has not been set up. The accessible studies in persons with type 1 diabetes in which low glycemic record eating methodologies were contrasted and high glycemic list diets (study length from 12 days to 6 weeks) don't give persuading proof regarding advantage. In subjects with type 2 diabetes, investigations of 2–12 weeks length of time looking at low glycemic list and high glycemic file diets report no steady upgrades in HbA1c, fructosamine, or insulin levels. The consequences for lipids from low glycemic list diets contrasted and high glycemic file weight control plans are blended.

In spite of the fact that it is clear that sugars do have varying glycemic reactions, the information uncover no unmistakable pattern in result advantages. If that there are long haul impacts on glycemia and lipids, these impacts have all the earmarks of being unassuming. Besides, the quantity of studies is constrained, and the outline and execution of a few of these studies are liable to feedback.

Fiber.

Concerning the all inclusive community, individuals with diabetes are urged to pick an assortment of fiber-containing foods, for example, entire grains, natural products, and vegetables, since they give vitamins, minerals, fiber, and different substances imperative for good wellbeing. Early fleeting studies utilizing a lot of fiber as a part of little quantities of subjects with type 1 diabetes recommended a constructive outcome on glycemia. Late studies have reported blended consequences for glycemia and lipids. In subjects with type 2 diabetes, it gives the idea that ingestion of a lot of fiber are important to give metabolic advantages on glycemic control, hyperinsulinemia, and plasma lipids. It is not clear whether the attractiveness and the gastrointestinal reactions of fiber in this sum would be adequate to a great many people.

Sweeteners.

The accessible proof from clinical studies exhibits that dietary sucrose does not increment glycemia more than isocaloric measures of starch. In this way, admission of sucrose and sucrose-containing foods by individuals with diabetes does not should be confined due to worry about disturbing hyperglycemia. Sucrose ought to be substituted for other starch sources in the food/dinner arrangement or, if added to the food/supper arrangement, satisfactorily secured with insulin or another glucose-bringing down medicine. Furthermore, admission of different supplements ingested with sucrose, for example, fat, should be considered.

In subjects with diabetes, fructose delivers a lower postprandial reaction when it replaces sucrose or starch in the eating routine; on the other hand, this advantage is tempered by worry that fructose might unfavorably impact plasma lipids. In this way, the utilization of included fructose as a sweetening specialists is not prescribed; nonetheless, there is no motivation to suggest that individuals with diabetes maintain a strategic distance from normally happening fructose in organic products, vegetables, and different foods. Therapeutic nutrition treatment is an essential segment of diabetes administration and of diabetes self-administration training. Yet numerous confusions exist concerning nutrition and diabetes. Additionally, in clinical practice, nutrition suggestions that have practically zero supporting proof have been are as yet being given to persons with diabetes. As needs be, this position proclamation gives proof based standards and suggestions for diabetes medicinal nutrition treatment. The method of reasoning for this position articulation is talked about in the American Diabetes Association specialized audit "Proof Based Nutrition Principles and Recommendations for the Treatment and Prevention of Diabetes and Related Complications," which examines in subtle element the distributed exploration for every standard and suggestion (1).

Verifiably, nutrition

Sugar alcohols create a lower postprandial glucose reaction than fructose, sucrose, or glucose and have lower accessible vitality values. Be that as it may, there is no confirmation that the sums liable to be devoured in a dinner or day result in a huge decrease altogether day by day vitality admission or change in long haul glycemia. The utilization of sugar alcohols gives off an impression of being protected; on the other hand, they might bring about loose bowels, particularly in kids.

The Food and Drug Administration has affirmed four non-nutritive sweeteners for use in the U.S.— saccharin, aspartame, acesulfame potassium, and sucralose. Before being permitted available, all experienced thorough examination and were appeared to be sheltered when devoured by general society, incorporating individuals with diabetes and during pregnancy.

Safe starch.

It has been suggested that foods containing normally happening safe starch (cornstarch) or foods changed to contain more safe starch (high amylose cornstarch) might adjust postprandial glycemic reaction, avert hypoglycemia, diminish hyperglycemia, and clarify contrasts in the glycemic record of a few foods. In any case, there are no distributed long haul concentrates on in subjects with diabetes to demonstrate advantage from the utilization of safe starch.

Foods containing starch from entire grains, organic products, vegetables, and low-fat milk ought to be incorporated into a sound eating regimen.

As to the glycemic impacts of starches, the aggregate sum of sugar in dinners or snacks is more imperative than the source or type. As sucrose does not expand glycemia to a more prominent degree than isocaloric measures of starch, sucrose and sucrose-containing foods don't should be limited by individuals with diabetes; be that as it may, they ought to be substituted for other sugar sources or, if included, secured with insulin or other glucose-bringing down pharmaceutical.

Non-nutritive sweeteners are protected when devoured inside of the adequate day by day consumption levels set up by the Food and Drug Administration.

B-Level confirmation

People getting serious insulin treatment ought to change their premeal insulin measurements taking into account the sugar substance of suppers.

Despite the fact that the utilization of low-glycemic list foods might decrease postprandial hyperglycemia, there is not adequate proof of long haul advantage to prescribe utilization of low-glycemic record diets as an essential system in food/supper arranging.

Likewise with the overall population, utilization of dietary fiber is to be empowered; be that as it may, there is no motivation to prescribe that individuals with diabetes expend a more noteworthy measure of fiber than different Americans.

C-Level proof

People accepting settled every day insulin measurements ought to attempt to be predictable in everyday sugar admission.

Master agreement

Starch and monounsaturated fat together ought to give 60–70% of vitality admission. On the other hand, the metabolic profile and requirement for weight reduction ought to be considered while deciding the monounsaturated fat substance of the eating regimen.

Sucrose and sucrose-containing foods ought to be eaten in the connection of a sound eating regimen.

PROTEIN AND DIABETES

In the U.S., protein consumption represents 15–20% of normal vitality admission, is genuinely predictable over all ages from early stages to more seasoned age, and seems, by all accounts, to be comparable in persons with diabetes. It has been accepted that in individuals with diabetes, variations from the norm of protein digestion system were less influenced by insulin lack and insulin resistance than glucose digestion system. Nonetheless, in subjects with type 2 diabetes, it has been exhibited that direct hyperglycemia can add to an greater turnover of protein, which proposes an greater requirement for protein. In subjects with type 1 diabetes treated with customary insulin treatment, transient dynamic studies have shown greater protein catabolism, recommending that close typical glycemia and a satisfactory protein admission are required. Since most grown-ups eat no less than half more protein than required, individuals with diabetes give off an impression of being ensured against protein malnutrition while devouring a standard eating regimen.

Dietary admission of protein is accounted for to be comparative in patients with or without nephropathy, however in all studies, protein admission was in the scope of normal admission and once in a while surpassed 20% of the vitality consumption. Admission of protein in the standard extent does not seem, by all accounts, to be connected with the improvement of diabetic nephropathy. On the other hand, the long haul impacts of devouring >20% of vitality as protein on the improvement of nephropathy has not been resolved, and thusly it might be reasonable to stay away from protein admissions >20% of aggregate every day vitality.

Various studies in sound subjects and in persons with controlled type 2 diabetes have shown that glucose from ingested protein does not show up in the general course, and hence protein does not build plasma glucose focuses. Moreover, the top glucose reaction to starch alone is like that of sugar and protein, proposing that protein does not moderate the assimilation of carb. In subjects with type 1 diabetes, the rate of reclamation of euglycemia after hypoglycemia, time to crest glucose levels, and resulting rate of glucose fall were comparable after treatment with either sugar alone or starch and protein.

The impacts of protein on regulation of vitality admission, satiety, and long haul weight reduction have not been satisfactorily examined. The long haul viability and security of high-protein low starch diets stays obscure.

In persons with controlled type 2 diabetes, ingested protein does not expand plasma glucose fixations, in spite of the fact that protein is generally as strong a stimulant of insulin emission as sugar. For persons with diabetes, particularly those not in ideal glucose control, the protein necessity might be more prominent than the Recommended Dietary Allowance, yet not more noteworthy than common admission.

For persons with diabetes, there is no proof to propose that typical protein admission (15–20% of aggregate every day vitality) ought to be altered if renal capacity is ordinary.

The long haul impacts of weight control plans high in protein and low in starch are obscure. Albeit such eating methodologies might create fleeting weight reduction and enhanced glycemia, it has not been set up that weight reduction is kept up long haul. The long haul impact of such weight control plans on plasma LDL cholesterol is likewise a worry.

DIETARY FAT AND DIABETES

Unsaturated fats and dietary cholesterol
The essential dietary fat objective in persons with diabetes is to constrain immersed fat and dietary cholesterol consumption. Soaked fat is the foremost dietary determinant of plasma LDL cholesterol. Moreover, persons with diabetes have all the earmarks of being more delicate to dietary cholesterol than the overall population.

In nondiabetic persons, low immersed fat and cholesterol diets diminish plasma all out cholesterol, LDL cholesterol, and triglycerides with blended impacts on HDL cholesterol. Positive relationships between's dietary aggregate and soaked fat and changes in plasma complete cholesterol and LDL and HDL cholesterol are watched. Including exercise results in more prominent abatements in plasma all out and LDL cholesterol and triglycerides and keeps the reduction in HDL cholesterol connected with low-fat eating methodologies. Be that as it may, thinks about in persons with diabetes showing impacts of particular rates of dietary soaked unsaturated fats and particular measures of dietary cholesterol are not accessible. Thusly, the objective for persons with diabetes continues as before concerning the overall public.

In metabolic study diets, in which vitality admission and weight are held consistent, slims down low in immersed fat and high in starch or advanced with cis-monounsaturated unsaturated fats (monounsaturated fat) lower plasma LDL cholesterol comparably. Low-soaked fat (i.e., 10% of vitality) high sugar diets increment postprandial levels of plasma glucose, insulin, triglycerides and, in a few studies, diminish plasma HDL cholesterol when contrasted in metabolic studies with isocaloric high monounsaturated fat eating methodologies. Notwithstanding, high-monounsaturated fat eating methodologies have not been appeared to enhance fasting plasma glucose or HbA1c values. There is worry that when such high monounsaturated fat eating regimens are eaten not indispensable outside of a controlled setting, it might bring about greater vitality allow and weight pick up. In this manner, both the metabolic profile and the need to get more fit will decide nutrition treatment suggestions. Moreover, ethnic or social.inclinations might assume a part in figuring out if immersed fat is to be supplanted with sugar or monounsaturated fat.

Polyunsaturated fats have not been very much concentrated on in persons with diabetes. At the point when contrasted and immersed fat, polyunsaturated fats seem to lower plasma all out and LDL cholesterol, however not and in addition monounsaturated fats. N-3 polyunsaturated unsaturated fat supplements have been appeared to lower plasma triglyceride levels in persons with type 2 diabetes.

Despite the fact that the going with ascend in plasma LDL cholesterol is of concern, glucose digestion system is not liable to be antagonistically influenced with their utilization. N-3 supplements might be most gainful in the treatment of extreme hypertriglyceridemia. While n-3 unsaturated fat studies in persons with diabetes have essentially utilized supplements, there is confirmation from the overall public that foods containing n-3 unsaturated fats have cardioprotective impacts. A few servings of fish for every week give dietary n-3 polyunsaturated fat and can be prescribed.

Real wellsprings of trans unsaturated fats in the eating routine incorporate items produced using halfway hydrogenated oils, for example, prepared items (counting saltines and other nibble foods), treats, doughnuts, breads, and items like fries or pan fried in hydrogenated shortening. Creature sources, including dairy items, give littler measures of trans unsaturated fats. The impact of trans unsaturated fats is like soaked fats in raising plasma LDL cholesterol. Also, trans unsaturated fats lower plasma HDL cholesterol. In this manner, admission of trans unsaturated fats ought to be restricted.

Plant sterol and stanol esters obstruct the intestinal assimilation of dietary and biliary cholesterol. Plant sterols/stanols in measures of ~2 g/day have been appeared to lower aggregate and LDL cholesterol.

Low-fat eating rgimen
In studies assessing the impact of not obligatory vitality admission as a component of dietary fat substance, low-fat high-starch eating regimens are connected with a transient diminishing in vitality consumption and unassuming weight reduction to another harmony body weight. With this unobtrusive weight reduction, a diminishing in

plasma complete cholesterol and triglycerides and an expansion in HDL cholesterol happen. Predictable with this, low-fat high-starch diets over drawn out stretches of time have demonstrated no expansion in plasma triglycerides and, when reported, small weight reduction.

Fat alternatives

Dietary fat admission can be decreased by bringing down the measure of high fat foods in the providing so as to eat regimen or lower-fat or without fat adaptations of food and refreshments or by utilizing fat replacers (fixings that copy the properties of fat yet with altogether less calories) in food plans. The Food and Drug Administration gives affirmation that present fat replacers/substitutes are sheltered to use in foods. General utilization of foods with fat replacers might decrease dietary fat admission (counting immersed fat and cholesterol), yet may not lessen downright vitality allow or weight. Long haul studies are expected to survey the impacts of foods containing fat replacers on vitality consumption and on the macronutrient substance of the eating regimens of individuals with diabetes.

Under 10% of vitality admission ought to be gotten from soaked fats. A few people (i.e., persons with LDL cholesterol ≥100 mg/dl) might profit by bringing immersed fat admission down to <7% of vitality admission.

Dietary cholesterol admission ought to be <300 mg/day. A few people (i.e., persons with LDL cholesterol ≥100 mg/dl) might profit by bringing dietary cholesterol down to <200 mg/day.

B-Level proof

To lower LDL cholesterol, vitality got from soaked fat can be decreased if weight reduction is alluring or supplanted with either starch or monounsaturated fat when weight reduction is not an objective.

Admission of trans unsaturated fats ought to be minimized.

Lessened fat eating methodologies when kept up long haul add to unobtrusive loss of weight and change in dyslipidemia.

A few servings of fish for each week give dietary n-3 polyunsaturated fat and can be suggested.

Polyunsaturated fat admission ought to be ~10% of vitality admission.

FOOD BALANCE AND OBESITY

On account of the impacts of corpulence on insulin resistance, weight reduction is an imperative restorative target for persons with type 2 diabetes. Transient studies have shown that weight reduction in subjects with type 2 diabetes is connected with diminished insulin resistance, enhanced measures of glycemia and dyslipidemia, and lessened pulse. In any case, long haul information evaluating the degree to which these enhancements can be kept up are not accessible. The reason long haul weight reduction is troublesome for the vast majority to achieve is most likely on the grounds that vitality consumption, vitality use and in this manner body weight are controlled by the focal sensory system. This regulation seems, by all accounts, to be affected by hereditary variables. Besides, ecological components regularly make shedding pounds troublesome for those hereditarily inclined to stoutness.

Proof shows that organized, escalated way of life projects including member instruction, individualized guiding, diminished dietary fat and vitality admission, normal physical movement, and incessant member contact are important to deliver long haul weight reduction of as much as 5–7% of beginning weight. At the point when counting calories to shed pounds, fat is likely the most essential supplement to confine. Unconstrained food utilization and downright vitality admission are greater when the eating routine is high in fat and diminished when the eating routine is low in fat. Exercise independent from anyone else has just a small impact on weight reduction. Be that as it may, practice is to be supported in light of the fact that it enhances insulin affectability, intensely brings down blood glucose, and is critical in long haul upkeep of weight reduction. Weight reduction with behavioral treatment alone likewise has been unobtrusive, and behavioral methodologies might be most helpful as an aide to other weight reduction procedures. Then again, ideal methodologies for anticipating and treating weight long haul have yet to be characterized.

Standard weight reduction diets give 500–1,000 less calories than evaluated to be essential for weight upkeep. Albeit numerous individuals can lose some weight (as much as 10% of starting weight) with such eating regimens, the therapeutic writing records that without alternate segments of a serious way of life project, long haul results are poor. The larger part of individuals recapture the weight they have lost.

Feast substitutions give a characterized measure of vitality frequently as a recipe item. Utilization of supper substitutions on more than one occasion day by day to supplant a standard feast can bring about critical weight reduction, yet dinner substitution treatment must be proceeded if weight reduction is to be kept up. Low calorie diets (VLCDs) give 800 or less calories day by day and produce generous weight reduction and quick changes in glycemia and lipemia in persons with type 2 diabetes.

At the point when VLCDs are halted and self-chose dinners are reintroduced, weight addition is normal. Along these lines, VLCDs seem to have restricted utility in the treatment of type 2 diabetes and ought to just be considered in conjunction with an organized weight upkeep program.

The accessible information propose that weight reduction pharmaceuticals might be helpful in the treatment of overweight persons with type 2 diabetes. On the other hand, their impact is small. Additionally, the accessible information propose that these meds just work the length of they are taken and ought to be utilized as a part of conjunction with way of life procedures. These medications ought to be utilized just as a part of individuals with BMI >27.0 kg/m2.

Albeit gastric diminishment surgery can be a powerful weight reduction treatment for extreme heftiness (counting serious stoutness in persons with type 2 diabetes), this surgery ought to just be considered for patients with a BMI ≥35 kg/m2. There are no information contrasting restorative and surgical methodologies with weight reduction, and in this way the relative advantages and dangers of surgical methodologies are unverifiable. In this way, gastric decrease surgery ought to be viewed as problematic in treating diabetes.

In insulin-safe people, diminished vitality admission and unobtrusive weight reduction enhance insulin resistance and glycemia in the short-term.

Organized projects that accentuate way of life changes, including training, diminished fat (<30% of every day vitality) and vitality admission, normal physical movement, and general member contact, can deliver long haul weight reduction on the request of 5–7% of beginning weight.

Exercise and conduct adjustment are most valuable as extras to other weight reduction methodologies. Activity is useful in upkeep of weight reduction.

Standard weight lessening diets, when utilized alone, are unrealistic to deliver long haul weight reduction. Organized escalated way of life projects are fundamental.

MICRONUTRIENTS AND DIABETES

Persons with diabetes ought to be taught about the significance of devouring satisfactory measures of vitamins and minerals from normal food sources and in addition the potential poisonous quality of megadoses of vitamin and mineral supplements. Albeit hard to discover, if inadequacies of vitamins and minerals are distinguished, supplementation can be advantageous. Select populaces, for example, the elderly, pregnant or lactating ladies, strict veggie lovers, and those on calorie-limited weight control plans, might profit by supplementation with a multivitamin arrangement.

Since diabetes might be a condition of greater oxidative anxiety, there has been enthusiasm for recommending cancer prevention agent vitamins to individuals with diabetes. By and large, megadoses of dietary cell reinforcements—vitamin C, vitamin E, selenium, beta carotene, and different carotenoids—have not showed security against cardiovascular illness, diabetes, or growth. Albeit substantial observational studies have demonstrated a connection between's dietary or supplemental utilization of cell reinforcements and cardiovascular advantage, huge fake treatment controlled trials have neglected to demonstrate an advantage and, in a few occasions, have proposed unfriendly impacts of cancer prevention agent vitamins. The part of folate in averting conception deformities is broadly acknowledged, however the part of folate supplementation to bring down homocysteine and to diminish cardiovascular occasions is not clear. The part of vitamins B1, B6, and B12 in the treatment of diabetic neuropathy has not been built up and can't be prescribed as a normal restorative alternative. The utilization of nicotinduringe to safeguard β-cell mass in recently determined subjects to have type 1 diabetes is under scrutiny; nonetheless, an advantageous impact has not been obviously illustrated.

Inadequacies of specific minerals, for example, potassium, magnesium, and conceivably zinc and chromium, might bother starch narrow mindedness. While the requirement for potassium or magnesium substitution is generally simple to identify taking into account low serum levels, the requirement for zinc or chromium supplementation is more hard to distinguish.

Advantageous impacts on glycemia from chromium supplementation have been accounted for. On the other hand, the populaces concentrated on might have had negligible benchmark chromium status, and in the biggest study, chromium status was not assessed either at pattern or taking after supplementation. Other very much composed studies have neglected to demonstrate any noteworthy advantage from chromium supplementation on glycemic control in individuals with diabetes. At the present, regale from chromium supplementation in persons with diabetes has not been indisputably illustrated.

A day by day admission of 1,000–1,500 mg of calcium, particularly in more established subjects with diabetes, is suggested. This proposal has all the earmarks of being sheltered and liable to lessen osteoporosis in more established persons. The estimation of calcium supplementation in more youthful persons is questionable.

The part of vanadium salts in diabetes has been investigated. There is no unmistakable proof of adequacy, and there is potential for danger. An assortment of home grown arrangements have been appeared to have unobtrusive valuable impacts on glycemia. In any case, economically accessible items are not all around institutionalized and differ extraordinarily in the substance of dynamic fixings. In persons with diabetes, there is no proof to propose long haul advantage from home grown arrangements. They likewise can possibly connect with drugs. In this manner, it is critical that medicinal services suppliers know when patients with diabetes are utilizing these items.

There is no reasonable confirmation of advantage from vitamin or mineral supplementation in individuals with diabetes who don't have basic lacks. Exemptions incorporate folate for aversion of conception deformities and calcium for counteractive action of bone malady.

There is no reasonable confirmation of advantage from vitamin or mineral supplementation in individuals with diabetes who don't have basic lacks. Exemptions incorporate folate for aversion of conception deformities and calcium for counteractive action of bone malady.

Routine supplementation of the eating regimen with cancer prevention agents is not informed on the grounds that concerning vulnerabilities identified with long haul adequacy and security.

Liquor AND DIABETES

For persons with diabetes, the same safety measures apply in regards to the utilization of liquor that apply to the all inclusive community. Abstention from liquor ought to be exhorted for ladies during pregnancy and for individuals with other restorative issues, for example, pancreatitis, propelled neuropathy, serious hypertriglyceridemia, or liquor misuse. If that people drink liquor, close to two liquor containing drinks for each day for grown-up men and close to one beverage for every day for grown-up ladies is prescribed. One beverage, or mixed drink, is generally characterized as 12 oz of brew, 5 oz of wine, or 1.5 oz of refined spirits, each of which contains ~15 g of liquor. The cardioprotective impacts of liquor show up not to be controlled by the type of mixed drink expended.

Liquor can have both hypoglycemic and hyperglycemic impacts in individuals with diabetes. These impacts are controlled by the measure of liquor intensely ingested, if overwhelmed by or without food and if use is perpetual and inordinate. In studies utilizing moderate measures of liquor ingested with food in individuals with type 1 or type 2 diabetes, liquor had no intense impact on blood glucose or insulin levels. In this way, mixed refreshments ought to be viewed as an expansion to the standard food/supper arrangement for all individuals with diabetes, and no food ought to be excluded.

Substantial or exorbitant liquor utilization is a main avoidable reason for death in the U.S. In any case, epidemiological confirmation in nondiabetic persons proposes that light-to-direct liquor ingestion in grown-ups is connected with greater insulin affectability and diminished danger of type 2 diabetes, coronary illness, and stroke. In grown-ups with diabetes, interminable admission of light-to-direct sums (5–15 g/day) was connected with diminished danger for coronary illness, probably because of the attendant increment in plasma HDL cholesterol. There gives off an impression of being a U-or J-formed relationship of liquor admission and circulatory strain. While light-to-direct measures of liquor don't raise circulatory strain, a solid affiliation exists between incessant over the top admission of liquor (>30–60 g/day) and pulse in men and ladies.

If that people drink liquor, every day admission ought to be restricted to one beverage for grown-up ladies and two beverages for grown-up men. One beverage is characterized as 12 oz of lager, 5 oz of wine, or 1.5 oz of refined spirits.

To decrease danger of hypoglycemia, liquor ought to be overwhelmed by food.

Unique CONSIDERATIONS FOR TYPE 1 DIABETES

Nutrition suggestions for a sound way of life for the overall population are additionally suitable for persons with type 1 diabetes. What contrasts for people requiring insulin is the reconciliation of an insulin regimen into their way of life. With the numerous insulin choices now accessible, a suitable insulin regimen can more often than not be produced to adjust to an individual's favored supper routine and food decisions. For persons accepting escalated insulin treatment, the aggregate starch substance of suppers (and snacks) is the real determinant of the premeal insulin dosage and postprandial glucose reaction. For persons getting altered insulin regimens and not conforming premeal insulin measurements, consistency of starch admission is suggested.

Enhanced glycemic control with insulin treatment is frequently connected with greater body weight. Due to the potential for weight increase to antagonistically influence glycemia, lipids, pulse, and general wellbeing, counteractive action of weight addition is alluring. In spite of the fact that the sugar substance of the supper decides the premeal insulin measurements, consideration ought to additionally be paid to aggregate vitality admission from protein and fat.

For arranged activity, lessening in insulin measurements might be the favored decision to anticipate hypoglycemia. Extra sugar might be required for impromptu work out. Moderate-power exercise builds glucose uptake by 2–3 mg · kg–1 · min–1 above regular necessities. In this way, a 70-kg individual would require 8.4–12.6 g (10–15) starch every hour of moderate physical action. More sugar would be required for extreme action .

Unique CONSIDERATIONS FOR TYPE 2 DIABETES

Nutrition suggestions for a sound way of life for the overall population are likewise fitting for persons with type 2 diabetes. Since numerous persons with type 2 diabetes are overweight and insulin safe, restorative nutrition treatment ought to accentuate way of life changes that outcome in diminished vitality allow and greater vitality consumption through physical action. Numerous individuals with diabetes additionally have dyslipidemia and hypertension, making decreases in dietary admission of soaked fat, cholesterol, and sodium attractive. In this manner, the accentuation of nutrition treatment for type 2 diabetes is on way of life procedures to lessen glycemia, dyslipidemia, and circulatory strain. These procedures ought to be actualized when the analysis of diabetes is made.

Greater physical action can prompt enhanced glycemia, diminished insulin resistance, and lessened cardiovascular danger variables. Division of food admission, three suppers or littler dinners and snacks, ought to be founded on individual inclinations. Treatment with insulin or insulin secretagogues requires consistency in timing of suppers and sugar content. Various insulin dosing regimens take into account a more adaptable food admission and way of life in persons with type 2 diabetes.

Therapeutic NUTRITION THERAPY FOR SPECIAL POPULATIONS
Nutrition proposals for kids and teenagers with type 1 diabetes ought to concentrate on accomplishing blood glucose objectives that keep up ordinary development and improvement without over the top hypoglycemia. This can be proficient through individualized food and dinner arranging, adaptable insulin regimens and calculations, self-blood glucose observing, and instruction advancing choice making taking into account results. Supplement prerequisites for youngsters and teenagers with type 1 or type 2 diabetes give off an impression of being like other same age kids and youths. Watchful thought of a tyke's craving must be utilized while deciding vitality prerequisites. The perfect system for assessing a youngster's or juvenile's vitality needs is a food/nutrition history of a commonplace every day consumption, giving that development and advancement are inside of ordinary breaking points. An assessment of weight addition and development starts at determination by recording tallness and weight on pediatric development diagrams. Sufficiency of vitality admission can be assessed by taking after weight pick up and development designs all the time.

Withholding food or having a youngster eat reliably without a hunger for food with an end goal to control blood glucose ought to be disheartened. Macronutrient creation of the nutrition solution ought to be individualized by glucose and plasma lipid objectives and prerequisites for development and advancement.

Nutrition proposals for youth with type 2 diabetes concentrates on treatment objectives to standardize glycemia and encourage a solid way of life (3). Fruitful treatment with nutrition treatment and physical movement can be characterized as discontinuance of extreme weight pick up with ordinary direct development and accomplishment of blood glucose objectives. Nutrition suggestions ought to additionally address related cardiovascular danger elements, for example, hypertension and dyslipidemia. Conduct alteration procedures to diminishing high-vitality high-fat food consumption while empowering good dieting propensities and normal physical action for the whole family ought to be considered.

Individualized food/dinner arrangements and concentrated insulin regimens can give adaptability to youngsters and teenagers with diabetes to suit sporadic feast times and plans, fluctuating hankering, and shifting movement levels.

Individualized food/feast arranges and serious insulin regimens can give adaptability to kids and youths with diabetes to suit sporadic dinner times and plans, fluctuating hankering, and differing action levels. Supplement prerequisites for kids and youths with type 1 or type 2 diabetes give off an impression of being like other same age youngsters and teenagers.

PREGNANCY AND LACTATION WITH DIABETES

The objectives of medicinal nutrition treatment for pregnancy are to give sufficient maternal and fetal nutrition, vitality consumption for proper weight pick up, and any important vitamin and mineral supplements. During pregnancy convoluted by diabetes, restorative nutrition treatment is additionally vital in accomplishing and keeping up ideal glycemic control.

Unless a lady starts pregnancy with drained body saves, vitality needs don't increment in the first trimester. An extra 300 kcal/day are recommended during the second and third trimester for expansions in maternal blood volume and increments in bosom, uterus and fat tissue, placental development, fetal development, and amniotic liquids. On the other hand, effective pregnancy results have been accounted for with lower vitality admissions.

Notwithstanding sufficient vitality admission, pregnant ladies need to eat a solid eating routine with satisfactory protein (0.75 g · kg−1 · day−1 in addition to an extra 10 g/day). Supplement necessity during pregnancy and lactation are comparative for ladies with and without diabetes. For all ladies who are equipped for getting to be pregnant, 400 µg/day of folic corrosive from strengthened foods and/or a supplement, and additionally food folate from an assortment of foods, is prescribed for the avoidance of neural tube deformities and other intrinsic irregularities. During pregnancy, a solid eating regimen bringing about proper weight pick up for the most part supplies all vitamins and minerals required. There is deficient confirmation to bolster pre-birth vitamin-mineral supplementation; on the other hand, they are regularly endorsed on account of instability of nutrition status and admission. Evaluation of the pregnant lady's eating examples might yield particular individual needs.

The Food and Drug Administration has endorsed four non-nutritive sweeteners, which are sheltered to use during pregnancy. Similarly as with nondiabetic ladies, ladies with diabetes ought to maintain a strategic distance from mixed drinks during pregnancy.

Pregnancy with earlier onset type 1 or type 2 diabetes

Prepregnancy nutrition treatment incorporates an individual pre-birth food/feast plan to advance blood glucose control. During pregnancy, the dissemination of the vitality allow and sugars in the dinner arrangement ought to be founded on the lady's food and dietary patterns, blood glucose records, and the normal physiological impacts of pregnancy on her body. Standard suppers and snacks are critical to maintain a strategic distance from hypoglycemia because of the persistent fetal draw of glucose from the mother. A night nibble is normally important to diminish the potential for overnight hypoglycemia and fasting ketosis. Blood glucose observing and every day food records give profitable data to insulin and feast arrangement alterations.

Gestational diabetes mellitus

Nutrition treatment for gestational diabetes advances nutrition for maternal and fetal wellbeing with sufficient vitality levels for proper gestational weight pick up, accomplishment and upkeep of normoglycemia, and nonappearance of ketones. Starch is disseminated for the duration of the day into three little to-direct measured dinners and 2–4 snacks. A night nibble might be expected to forestall quickened ketosis overnight. Starch is by and large less very much endured at breakfast than at different dinners. Particular nutrition and food suggestions are resolved and adjusted in light of individual evaluation and self-blood glucose checking information.

Vitality admission ought to accommodate an alluring weight pick up during pregnancy. Hypocaloric diets in large ladies with gestational diabetes result in ketonemia and ketonuria. A more unobtrusive vitality limitation (30% calorie-confinement of assessed vitality needs) seems to decrease mean blood glucose levels without rise in plasma free unsaturated fats or ketonuria. Every day food records, week by week weight checks, and ketone testing can be utilized to decide singular vitality proposals and whether a lady is undereating to keep away from insulin treatment.

General oxygen consuming activity has been appeared to lower fasting and postprandial glucose focuses and might be utilized as a subordinate to nutrition treatment to enhance maternal glycemia. There is inadequate confirmation to suggest a particular type of activity. Blood glucose information are important to assess the adequacy of nutrition treatment, exercise, and the requirement for pharmacological treatment. If that insulin treatment is added to nutrition treatment, keeping up starch consistency at suppers and snacks to encourage insulin modification turns into an essential objective.

Albeit most ladies with gestational diabetes return to ordinary glucose resilience baby blues, they are at greater danger of creating gestational diabetes in consequent pregnancies and type 2 diabetes further down the road. Way of life changes went for decreasing or counteracting weight pick up and expanding physical movement after pregnancy is prescribed and can lessen the danger of resulting diabetes.

Lactation

Breastfeeding is suggested for ladies with previous diabetes or gestational diabetes; on the other hand, fruitful lactation requires arranging and coordination of consideration. Breastfeeding brings down blood glucose, regularly requiring insulin-treated ladies to eat a nibble containing starch either before or during breastfeeding. Vitality necessities during the initial 6 months of lactation require an extra ~200 calories over the pregnancy feast arrangement. On the other hand, a vitality admission of ~1,800 kcal/day as a rule meets the nutritional prerequisites for lactation and might consider a progressive weight reduction.

Nutrition necessities during pregnancy and lactation are comparative for ladies with and without diabetes. Therapeutic nutrition treatment for gestational diabetes concentrates on food decisions for fitting weight pick up, normoglycemia, and nonattendance of ketones.

For a few ladies with gestational diabetes, unobtrusive vitality and sugar confinement might be proper. There is restricted examination on changing nutritional needs with maturing and for all intents and purposes none in subjects with diabetes. In this way, nutrition proposals for more established grown-ups with diabetes must be extrapolated from what is known from the overall public. The most solid pointer of poor nutritional status in the elderly is presumably an adjustment in body weight. When all is said in done, automatic addition or loss of >10 pounds or 10% body weight in <6 months shows a need to assess if the reason is nutrition-related.

The requirement for weight reduction in overweight more established grown-ups ought to be deliberately assessed. More established individuals with diabetes, particularly those in long haul care offices, have a tendency to be underweight instead of overweight. Low body weight has been connected with more prominent grimness and mortality in this age bunch.

Exercise preparing can essentially diminish the decrease in maximal high-impact limit (Vo2) that happens with age, enhance hazard variables for atherosclerosis, moderate the decrease in age-related incline body mass, diminish focal adiposity, and enhance insulin affectability; all of which is useful for the more established grown-up with diabetes.

A day by day multivitamin supplement might be fitting for more seasoned grown-ups, particularly those with decreased vitality admission. Every single more seasoned grown-up ought to be informed to have a calcium admission with respect to no less than 1,200 mg day by day.

The inconvenience of dietary confinements on elderly inhabitants with diabetes in long haul wellbeing offices is not justified. Malnutrition and drying out might create as a result of absence of food decisions, low quality of food, and superfluous limitations. Particular diabetic weight control plans don't give off an impression of being better than standard (normal) diets in such settings. Subsequently, it is suggested that occupants are served the general (unhindered) menu with consistency in the sum and timing of sugar. There is no confirmation to bolster weight control plans, for example, "no concentrated desserts" or "no sugar included," which are frequently served to the elderly in long haul care offices. Moreover, it might frequently be desirable over roll out drug improvements to control blood glucose than to actualize food confinements. Vitality prerequisites for more seasoned grown-ups are not exactly for more youthful grown-ups.

Physical movement ought to be supported.

In the elderly, undernutrition is more probable than overnutrition, and subsequently alert ought to be practiced when recommending weight reduction diets.

Restorative NUTRITION THERAPY FOR THE TREATMENT/PREVENTION OF ACUTE COMPLICATIONS OF DIABETES AND CO-MORBID CONDITIONS Acute confusions Hypoglycemia.

Changes in food consumption, physical action, and medication(s) can add to the improvement of hypoglycemia. Treatment of hypoglycemia requires ingestion of glucose or starch containing foods. The intense glycemic reaction corresponds preferred with the glucose content over with the sugar substance of the food. With insulin-prompted hypoglycemia, 10 g of oral glucose can raise blood glucose levels by ~40 mg/dl (2.2 mmol/l) more than 30 min, and 20 g of oral glucose can raise blood glucose levels by ~60 mg/dl (3.3 mmol/l) more than 45 min. For every situation, glucose levels start to fall at ~60 min after glucose ingestion (4).

Albeit immaculate glucose might be the favored treatment, any type of sugar that contains glucose will raise blood glucose. Adding protein to the sugar treatment of hypoglycemia does not influence the glycemic reaction and does not avert ensuing hypoglycemia. Including fat, notwithstanding, might impede the intense glycemic reaction. During hypoglycemia, gastric exhausting rates are twice as high as during euglycemia and are comparable for fluids and for strong foods.

Intense ailment in persons with type 1 diabetes can build the danger for diabetic ketoacidosis. During intense sickness the requirement for insulin proceeds. Besides, related greater levels of counterregulatory hormones might build insulin prerequisites. Testing blood glucose, testing blood or pee for ketones, drinking satisfactory measures of liquid, and ingesting starch, particularly if blood glucose level is <100 mg/dl (5.5 mmol/l), are vital during an intense ailment. In grown-ups, ingestion of ~150–200 g sugar day by day (45–50 g, or three to four starch decisions, each 3–4 h) ought to be adequate, alongside prescription changes, to keep glucose in the objective reach and to avert starvation ketosis.

Glucose is the favored treatment for hypoglycemia, albeit any type of sugar that contains glucose might be utilized.

Ingestion of 15–20 g of glucose is a viable treatment, yet blood glucose might just be briefly adjusted. During intense sicknesses, testing blood glucose and blood or pee for ketones, drinking sufficient measures of liquids, and ingesting starch are imperative.

Starting reaction to treatment for hypoglycemia ought to be seen in ~10–20 min; be that as it may, blood glucose ought to be assessed again in ~60 min, as extra treatment might be essential.

HYPERTENSION

Restorative nutrition treatment for the administration of hypertension has concentrated on weight diminishment and lessening sodium admission. Different variables that have been considered incorporate liquor, potassium, calcium, and diet sythesis (complete fat, immersed fat, and cholesterol). A low-fat eating routine that incorporates foods grown from the ground (five to nine servings/day) and low-fat dairy items (two to four servings/day) will be rich in potassium, magnesium, and calcium and unobtrusively decrease circulatory strain. There are few studies done only in subjects with diabetes. Reaction to sodium decrease might be more noteworthy in subjects who are "salt delicate," a component that might apply to numerous people with diabetes. At present, there is no accessible routine clinical measure to recognize persons who might be salt delicate. A few meta-investigations and surveys have reported the relationship between sodium allow and pulse. The mean impact of a moderate sodium confinement is accounted for to be a lessening of ~5 mmHg for systolic and ~2 mmHg for diastolic circulatory strain in hypertensive subjects and a decrease of ~3 mmHg for systolic and ~1 mmHg for diastolic pulse in normotensive subjects. Three levels of sodium admission were thought about in an eating routine containing natural products, vegetables, and low-fat dairy items and low altogether fat, immersed fat, and cholesterol. The lower the sodium allow, the more prominent the bringing down of circulatory strain (5).

There is a general relationship in individuals with diabetes between weight lessening and a diminishment in circulatory strain, yet there is incredible variability in the reaction. Decrease in circulatory strain can happen with a small measure of weight reduction.

A relationship between high liquor admission (≥3 drinks/day) and lifted circulatory strain has been accounted for; be that as it may, there is no significant contrast in pulse between individuals who expend <3 drinks/day and nondrinkers.

Clinical trials have reported a valuable impact of potassium supplementation on bringing down circulatory strain, though prove for a helpful impact from calcium and magnesium supplementation are deficient.

In both normotensive and hypertensive people, a lessening in sodium consumption brings down circulatory strain.

A small measure of weight reduction gainfully influences circulatory strain.

The objective ought to be to decrease sodium admission to 2,400 mg (100 mmol) or sodium chloride (salt) to 6,000 mg/day.

DYSLIPIDEMIA

Dyslipidemia (unusual lipid levels, lipoprotein arrangement, or both) is regularly found in persons with type 1 and type 2 diabetes. For most people with type 1 diabetes, powerful insulin treatment typically returns lipid levels to ordinary and more often than not brings down plasma triglycerides. Plasma LDL cholesterol might diminish unobtrusively also.

In grown-up people with raised plasma LDL cholesterol, immersed unsaturated fats ought to be restricted to <10% and ideally to <7% of vitality admission. Admissions of trans unsaturated fats ought to be restricted. If that soaked fat is supplanted, it can be supplanted with either starches or monounsaturated fats. Plasma LDL cholesterol bringing down can be improved by the expansion of plant stanols/sterols and by an expansion in solvent (thick) fiber.

Fat persons with type 1 diabetes and numerous persons with type 2 diabetes show a dyslipidemia with greater plasma triglycerides, lessened HDL cholesterol, and little thick LDL particles that holds on in spite of enhanced glycemic control. This dyslipidemia is firmly connected with greater body adiposity that is abdominally (instinctively) disseminated. For these persons, suggested way of life changes incorporate 1) decreasing soaked fat to <7% of vitality and dietary cholesterol to <200 mg/day, 2) expanding thick (solvent) fiber (10–25 g/day) and plant stanols/sterols (2 g/day) to improve plasma LDL cholesterol bringing down, 3) small weight reduction, and 4) greater physical action. Dietary fat confinement and weight reduction will prompt diminished plasma triglycerides and a small bringing down of plasma LDL cholesterol. Supplanting soaked fat with sugar has been appeared by most, however not all, studies to bring about enhancements in plasma LDL cholesterol with useful or impartial consequences for plasma triglycerides. Monounsaturated fat can likewise be substituted for immersed fat. On the other hand, expanding dietary fat can prompt an expansion in vitality allow and weight pick up. Normal physical action will likewise diminish plasma triglycerides and enhance insulin affectability.

For patients with tirelessly lifted plasma triglycerides regardless of the expansion of prescription, supplementation with fish oils that incorporate n-3 unsaturated fats might be suggested. On the other hand, fish oils might build plasma LDL cholesterol, so observing is required. Patients with plasma triglycerides >1,000 mg/dl are at greater danger for chylomicronemia disorder and pancreatitis and ought to have limitation of a wide range of dietary fat and establishment of lipid-bringing down pharmaceutical.

For persons with raised plasma LDL cholesterol, soaked unsaturated fats and trans-immersed unsaturated fats ought to be restricted to <10% and maybe to <7% of vitality.

For persons with raised plasma triglycerides, decreased HDL cholesterol, and little thick LDL cholesterol (the metabolic disorder), enhanced glycemic control, unassuming weight reduction, dietary soaked fat limitation, greater physical movement, and consolidation of monounsaturated fats might be valuable.

Vitality got from immersed fat can be decreased if weight reduction is alluring or supplanted with either starches or monounsaturated fats if weight reduction is not an objective. NEPHROPATHY

A few dietary variables have been recognized as having a part in the avoidance of nephropathy. In persons with type 1 or type 2 diabetes who have microalbuminuria, even little decreases in protein admission have been appeared to enhance glomerular filtration rate and to lessen urinary egg whites discharge rates. Concentrates on in subjects with type 1 diabetes and macroalbuminuria (clear nephropathy) demonstrated an abating of the decrease in glomerular filtration rate with dietary protein lessening to $0.8\,g \cdot kg-1 \cdot day-1$. In any case, such decreases ought to consider the need to keep up great nutritional status in patients with ceaseless renal disappointment. Protein limitation and other renal illness supper arrangements ought to be planned by an enrolled dietitian acquainted with restorative nutrition treatment for diabetes.

A few studies have investigated the potential advantage of plant protein instead of creature protein in renal deficiency. Long haul clinical trials are required in subjects with diabetes and nephropathy to figure out if ingestion of or decreases in specific types of protein have a useful impact.

In people with microalbuminuria, lessening of protein to 0.8–1.0 g · kg–1 · body wt–1per day and in people with plain nephropathy, diminishment to 0.8 g · kg–1 · body wt–1 every day might moderate the movement of nephropathy.

CATABOLIC ILLNESS

Catabolic illness states result in an adjustment in body compartments that might be portrayed by an greater extracellular liquid compartment (as often as possible with a real increment in body weight) and a related shrinkage of muscle to fat quotients and body cell mass. The size of late weight reduction, considering the vicinity of abundance liquid alongside the vicinity or nonappearance of clinical markers of anxiety and the measure of time the patient will be not able eat, ought to decide the requirement for nutrition mediation. A late weight reduction in overabundance of 10% requires an exhaustive nutrition evaluation. Unexpected weight reduction of 10–20% recommends moderate protein-calorie malnutrition, while lost >20% for the most part shows serious malnutrition.

A standard enteral recipe (half starch) or a lower-sugar (33–40% starch) equation might be utilized as a part of people with diabetes. Watchful observing of fundamental signs, hemodynamic information, weight, liquid equalization, plasma glucose and electrolytes, and corrosive based status is crucial. Meds, for the most part insulin, might should be conformed to keep up glycemic control. The necessities of most hospitalized patients can be met by giving 25–35 kcal/kg body wt. Consideration ought to be taken not to overload since this can fuel hyperglycemia, cause anomalous liver capacity, and expand oxygen utilization and carbon dioxide creation. Protein needs are ~1.0 g · kg–1 · body wt–1 for somewhat focused on patients and 1.5 g/kg for respectably to seriously focused on patients with typical hepatic and renal capacity. No less than 30% of aggregate vitality ought to be given as lipids.

The vitality needs of most hospitalized patients can be met by giving 25–35 kcal/kg body wt.

Protein needs are somewhere around 1.0 and 1.5 g/kg body wt; the higher end of the reach being for more focused on patients.

DIABETES PREVENTION

The significance of aversion of diabetes in high-hazard people is highlighted by the considerable and overall increment in the predominance of diabetes as of late. Hereditary vulnerability seems to assume a capable part if of type 2 diabetes in specific populaces. On the other hand, given that populace quality pools move gradually, the present plague likely reflects stamped changes in way of life. Way of life changes that are portrayed by diminished physical action and greater vitality utilization have together advanced corpulence, which is a solid danger component for diabetes that itself is impacted by both qualities and conduct. Notwithstanding the trouble in keeping up a decreased body weight long haul, a few studies have shown the potential for moderate managed weight reduction to considerably diminish the danger for type 2 diabetes. Clinical trial information from both the U.S. also, Finland now emphatically bolster the potential for moderate weight reduction to decrease the danger for diabetes (6,7). A dynamic way of life additionally has been shown in various planned studies to avoid or defer the improvement of type 2 diabetes. Both moderate and lively practice diminish danger of impeded glucose resilience and type 2 diabetes.

Diminished admission of aggregate fat, especially immersed fat, might decrease hazard for diabetes. Greater diabetes rate is accounted for with greater admission of dietary fat, autonomous of aggregate calories, despite the fact that this impact is not showed in all studies. It creates the impression that a wide range of dietary fat (aside from n-3 unsaturated fats) might adversy affect insulin affectability. Soaked fat might have the best impact. Greater admission of polyunsaturated fat, in the connection of fitting aggregate vitality consumption for weight administration, might decrease the danger for type 2 diabetes.

Late studies have given proof to diminished danger of diabetes with greater admission of entire grains and dietary fiber. Albeit chose micronutrients might influence glucose and insulin digestion system, information to archive their part in the advancement of diabetes are meager or conflicting. Moderate liquor admission has been identified with enhanced insulin affectability and diminished danger for diabetes. On the other hand, deficient information exist to bolster a particular suggestion for moderate liquor consumption for anticipation of type 2 diabetes.

No nutritional proposals can be made for counteractive action of type 1 diabetes. Breastfeeding might be useful. Albeit expanding weight in youth might be identified with an expansion in the commonness of type 2 diabetes, especially in minority young people, there is deficient information at present to warrant a particular suggestions for avoidance of type 2 diabetes in youth. Greater physical movement, diminished vitality and fat admission, and resultant weight to be good.

Home Remedies for Diabetes

Diabetes, likewise called diabetes mellitus, has turned into an exceptionally regular heath issue. There are two fundamental types of diabetes-type 1 diabetes in which the body does not deliver insulin and type 2 diabetes in which the body does not create enough insulin or the insulin that is created does not work appropriately.

diabetes graph

A percentage of the normal indications of diabetes incorporate weakness, weight reduction (despite the fact that you are eating more), over the top thirst, greater pee, cut and wounds that are moderate to mend and obscured vision.

While there is no cure for diabetes, with your glucose level under control you can carry on with an absolutely typical life. There are different characteristic solutions for diabetes that will offer you some assistance with controlling your glucose level.

Supported connections

Home Remedies for Diabetes

Here are the main 10 home solutions for diabetes. Obviously, you additionally need to counsel a specialist for legitimate finding and treatment.

(Out of the 10, we have secured 3 very viable home cures in this video also.)

1. Biting Gourd

Biting gourd, otherwise called astringent melon, can be useful for controlling diabetes because of its blood glucose bringing down impacts. It tends to impact the glucose digestion system everywhere on your body as opposed to a specific organ or tissue.

It increments pancreatic insulin emission and counteracts insulin resistance. Consequently, sharp gourd is useful for both type 1 and type 2 diabetes. On the other hand, it can't be utilized to totally supplant insulin treatment.

Drink some astringent gourd juice on a vacant stomach every morning. Initially evacuate the seeds of a few biting gourds and utilize a juicer to extricate the juice. Include some water and after that drink it. Take after this treatment day by day in the morning for no less than two months.

Additionally, you can incorporate one dish made of astringent gourd day by day in your eating regimen.

2. Cinnamon

Powdered cinnamon can stimulating so as to bring down glucose levels insulin action. It contains bioactive segments that can forestall and battle diabetes.

Certain trials have demonstrated that it can fill in as a powerful alternative to lower glucose levels in instances of uncontrolled type-2 diabetes.

Cinnamon, nonetheless, ought not be taken in abundance because we ordinarily utilize Cassia cinnamon (found in most supermarkets) which contains a compound called coumarin. It is a lethal exacerbate that expands the danger of liver harm.

There is another assortment of this herb known as Ceylon cinnamon or "genuine cinnamon." It is considered more secure for wellbeing yet its consequences for blood glucose levels have not been concentrated satisfactorily.

Blend one-half to one teaspoon of cinnamon in some warm water. Drink it every day.

Another choice is to bubble two to four cinnamon sticks in some water and permit it to soak for 20 minutes. Drink this arrangement day by day until you see change. You can likewise add cinnamon to warm refreshments, smoothies and prepared products.

3. Fenugreek

Fenugreek is a herb that can likewise be utilized to control diabetes, enhance glucose resistance and lower glucose levels because of its hypoglycaemic movement. It additionally fortifies the discharge of glucose-ward insulin. Being high in fiber, it backs off the ingestion of starches and sugars.

Splash two tablespoons of fenugreek seeds in water overnight. Drink the water alongside the seeds in the morning on a void stomach. Take after this cure without come up short for a couple of months to cut down your glucose level.

Another alternative is to eat two tablespoons of powdered fenugreek seeds day by day with milk.

4. Indian Gooseberry (Amla)

Indian gooseberry, otherwise called Amla, is rich in vitamin C and Indian gooseberry juice advances legitimate working of your pancreas. Take a few Indian gooseberries, evacuate the seeds and granulate it into a fine glue. Put the glue in a fabric and press out the juice. Blend two tablespoon of the juice in some water and drink it every day on an unfilled stomach.

Then again, blend one tablespoon of Indian gooseberry juice in some biting gourd squeeze and drink it every day for a couple of months.

5. Dark Plum or Indian Black Berry (Jambul)

Dark plum or jambul, otherwise called jamun can offer a great deal in controlling blood some assistance with sugaring level because it contains anthocyanins, ellagic corrosive, hydrolysable tannins and so on.

Every part of the Jambul plant, for example, the leaves, berry and seeds can be utilized by those agony from diabetes. Truth be told, research has demonstrated that the products of the soil of this plant have hypoglycemic impacts as they decrease blood and pee sugar levels quickly.

The seeds, specifically, contain glycoside jamboline and alkaloid jambosine that manage control glucose levels. At whatever point this occasional organic product is accessible in the business sector, attempt to incorporate it in your eating routine as it can be extremely successful for the pancreas. Else you can make a powder of dried seeds of Jambul leafy foods this powder with water twice per day. This organic product is local to India and its neighboring nations yet you can discover it at Asian markets and natural shops.

6. Mango Leaves

The fragile and delicate mango leaves can be utilized to treat diabetes by directing insulin levels in the blood. They can likewise enhance blood lipid profiles. Drench 10 to 15 delicate mango leaves in a glass of water overnight. In the morning, channel the water and drink it on a void stomach.

You can likewise dry the leaves in the shade and granulate them. Eat one-half teaspoon of powdered mango leaves two times everyday.

Numerous regular herbs and flavors are asserted to have glucose bringing down properties that make them helpful for individuals with or at high danger of type 2 diabetes.

Various clinical studies have been completed as of late that show potential connections between home grown treatments and enhanced blood glucose control, which has prompted an expansion in individuals with diabetes utilizing these more "common" fixings to deal with their condition.

What home grown treatments are accessible?

Plant-based treatments that have been appeared in a few studies to have hostile to diabetic properties include:

Aloe vera

Bilberry remove

Sharp melon

Cinnamon

Fenugreek

Ginger

Okra

While such treatments are generally utilized as a part of ayurvedic and oriental prescription for regarding genuine conditions, for example, diabetes, numerous wellbeing specialists in the west stay distrustful about their reported health advantages.

Truth be told, because certain herbs, vitamins and supplements might interface with diabetes medicines (counting insulin) and build their hypoglycemic impacts, it is frequently contended that utilization of common treatments could decrease blood sugars to hazardously low levels and raise the danger of different diabetes intricacies.

Whatever your expected purposes behind utilizing these particular herbs, you should dependably talk about your arrangements with your specialist and diabetes medicinal services group first to guarantee they are alright for your condition and decide a suitable measurement.

Further natural treatments

The herbs and plant subordinates recorded underneath have been utilized customarily by local individuals in the treatment of diabetes, in the zones in which they develop. Numerous experience the ill effects of a lacking information base.

Allium

Allium sativum is all the more ordinarily known as garlic, and is thought to offer cancer prevention agent properties and smaller scale circulatory impacts. Albeit few studies have specifically connected allium with insulin and blood glucose levels, results have been certain.

Allium might cause a lessening in blood glucose, build emission and moderate the corruption of insulin. Constrained information is accessible be that as it may, and promote trials are required.

Bauhinia forficata and Myrcia uniflora

Bauhinia forficata develops in South America, and is utilized as a part of Brazilian home grown cures. This plant has been alluded to as 'vegetable insulin'. Myrcia uniflora is likewise generally utilized in South America. Thinks about using the herbs as tea implantations recommend that their hypoglycaemic impacts are exaggerated.

Coccinia indica

Coccinia indica is otherwise called the 'ivy gourd' and develops wild over the Indian subcontinent. Customarily utilized in ayurverdic cures, the herb has been found to contain insulin-mimetic properties (i.e; it copies the capacity of insulin).

Noteworthy changes in glycaemic control have been accounted for in studies including coccinia indica, and specialists trust that it ought to be concentrated further.

Ficus carica

Ficus carica, or fig-leaf, is understood as a diabetic cure in Spain and South-western Europe, however its dynamic segment is obscure. A few studies on creatures recommend that fig-leaf encourages glucose uptake.

The viability of the plant is, be that as it may, at present yet to be approved in the treatment of diabetes.

Ginseng

Ginseng is an aggregate name for an assortment of various plant species.

In a few studies using American ginseng, diminishes in fasting blood glucose were accounted for. Assortments incorporate Korean ginseng, Siberian ginseng, American ginseng and Japanese ginseng.

In a few fields the plant, especially the panax species, are hailed as 'cure-all.' As is the situation with a hefty portion of the herbs utilized far and wide in the treatment of diabetics, further long haul studies are expected to confirm the adequacy of ginseng.

Gymnema sylvestre

Gymnema sylvestre is likewise utilized in conventional ayurverdic pharmaceutical. The plant develops in the tropical woods of southern and focal India, and has been connected with critical blood glucose bringing down. A few studies in creatures have even reported recovery of islet cells and an expansion in beta-cell capacity.

Momordica charantia

Momordica Charantia goes under an assortment of names and is local to a few regions of Asia, India, Africa and South America. Advertised as charantia, it is otherwise called karela or karolla and intense melon. The herb might be arranged in an assortment of various ways, and might have the capacity to help diabetics with insulin emission, glucose oxidation and different procedures.

Intense impacts on blood glucose levels have likewise been accounted for.

Ocimum sanctum

Ocimum sanctum is a herb utilized in customary ayurverdic rehearses, and is generally known as heavenly basil. A controlled clinical trial demonstrated a constructive outcome on postprandial and fasting glucose, and specialists foresee that the herb could improve the working of beta cells, and encourage the insulin emission process.

Opuntia streptacantha

Opuntia streptacantha (nopal) is generally known as the thorny pear desert plant in the bone-dry locales where it develops.

Tenants of the Mexican desert have customarily utilized the plant in glucose control. Intestinal glucose uptake might be influenced by a few properties of the plant, and creature ponders have discovered critical declines in postprandial glucose and HbA1c.

By and by, to accept the thorny pear desert flora as a successful method for supporting diabetic patients, long haul clinical trials are required.

Silibum marianum

Silibum marianum is otherwise called milk thorn, and is an individual from the aster crew. Silymarin contains high groupings of flavinoids and cancer prevention agents, some of which might beneficially affect insulin resistance. The part of milk thorn in glycaemic control is minimal caught on.

Trigonella foenum graecum

Trigonella foenum graecum is known as fenugreek and is broadly developed in India, North Africa, and parts of the Mediterranean.

It is additionally a piece of Ayurverdic treatment, and is utilized broadly as a part of cooking.

Of the few non-controlled trials that have been completed on type 2 diabetics, most report enhanced glycaemic control. Further study is positively justified.

Further herbs that have been concentrated on, and might have beneficial outcomes for diabetic patients include:

Berberine

Cinnamomym tamala

Curry

Eugenia jambolana

Gingko

Phyllanthus amarus

Pterocarpus marsupium

Solanum torvum and

Vinca rosea

One purported 'serious sickness' that distresses a huge number of individuals around the globe is type 1 diabetes. Not at all like type 2 diabetes, where the body gets to be impervious to its own insulin, type 1 is described by the powerlessness of the body to sufficiently deliver insulin, as the beta cells inside of the pancreas which are in charge of the creation of insulin (and the proinsulin from which it is made) are either annihilated or truly debilitated. This can happen because of immune system issues, bacterial or viral diseases, contrary sustenances in the eating regimen and substance exposures (or a mix of any one or a greater amount of these elements), to give some examples real triggers.

But then, a lot of associate surveyed and distributed research now demonstrates that plant mixes, including numerous found inside generally expended nourishments, are equipped for invigorating beta cell recovery inside of the pancreas, and thus might be conceivably give a cure – really a four letter word, similarly as the benefit based model of solution goes, which flourishes with the idea of the seriousness of the sickness beset human body for manifestation administration.

The disclosure of the beta cell regenerative capability of different sustenance and mixes will undoubtedly steamed a thriving diabetes industry, with a large number of dollars of open and private cash consistently being filled raising money endeavors for a future "cure"; A cure that will probably be conveyed through the restrictively costly pharmaceutical,vaccine or biologic (e.g. undifferentiated cells, islet cell xenotransplantation) pipeline, which by the very way of the FDA drug endorsement process requires the advancement of manufactured (and along these lines patentable) mixes over normal ones.

We should examine the most recent preclinical study on the theme, distributed a month ago in the Canadian Journal of Physiology and Pharmacology[1]. A dynamic division of flaxseed, which analysts named Linun usitassimum dynamic portion (LU6), was found to produce an extensive variety of advantages in a type 1 diabetes creature model, including the accompanying:

Enhanced glucose use in the liver

Upheld standardized glycogenesis (glucose framing movement) in the liver and muscle tissue

Diminished pancreatic and intestinal glucosidase inhibitory action, which interprets into lower post-feast glucose heights

Considerably more wonderful was the perception that this flaxseed compound standardized plasma insulin and C-peptide levels (C peptide is not C-receptive protein, rather it is an immediate pointer of the amount of insulin is being delivered by the beta cells in the body. Take in more), a sign that beta cell capacity was adequately restored. The scientists portrayed the genuinely astounding results as takes after:

Standardization of plasma insulin and C-peptide levels were seen in diabetic mice, showing endogenous insulin discharge after the treatment with LU6. The histochemical and immunohistochemical investigation on pancreatic islets recommends the part of LU6 portion in islet recovery and insulin emission as obvious in expansion practical pancreatic islets creating insulin. Moreover, critical insulin delivering islet arrangement was additionally seen in vitro PANC-1 cells after LU6 treatment, showing the phone totals to be recently shaped islets. This recommends the capability of LU6 part in the development of new islets in vitro, and in addition in vivo. In this manner, LU6 can be utilized as a nutraceutical-based first-line treatment for diabetes. [emphasis added]

Remember this is not the first occasion when that flaxseed has been found to enhance glucose issue. We have a couple concentrates on GreenMedInfo.com as of now ordered on the theme that you can see here: Flaxseed and Diabetes.

Moreover, we have found a wide scope of common substances tentatively affirmed to empower beta cell recovery, 10 of which are recorded underneath:

Arginine: a recent report found that the amino corrosive L-arginine is fit for empowering the genesis of beta cells in a creature model of alloxan-instigated diabetes.

Avocado: A recent report found that avocado seed extricate diminished glucose in diabetic rats. Scientists watched a helpful and defensive impact on pancreatic islet cells in the treated gathering.

Berberine: A recent report found this plant compound, ordinarily found in herbs, for example, barberry and goldenseal, instigates beta cell recovery in diabetic rats, which loans clarification for why it has been utilized for a long time as a part of China to treat diabetes.

Chard: A recent report found that chard remove given to diabetic rats animates the recuperation of harmed beta cells.

Corn Silk: A recent report found that corn silk diminishes glucose and invigorates beta cell recovery in type 1 diabetic rats.

Curcumin (from Turmeric): A recent report found that curcumin invigorates beta cell recovery in type 1 diabetic rats. Moreover, a recent report found that curcumin jelly pancreatic islet cell survival and transplantation proficiency.

Genistein (from soy, red clover): A recent report found that genistein affects pancreatic beta-cell multiplication through actuation of various flagging pathways and forestalls insulin-lacking diabetes in mice.

Nectar: A 2010 human study found that long haul utilization of nectar may effectsly affect the metabolic confusions of type 1 diabetes, including conceivable beta cell recovery as demonstrating by expansions in fasting C-peptide levels.

Nigella Sativa (dark seed): A 2003 creature study found that dark seed utilization lead to halfway recovery/multiplication of the beta-cells.[11] A 2010 human concentrate likewise found that the utilization of one gram of dark seed a day for up to 12 weeks had an expansive scope of advantageous impacts in diabetics, including expanding beta cell capacity.

Stevia: A 2011 human study found that stevia has hostile to diabetic properties, including renewing harmed beta cells, and contrasts positively and the medication glibenclduringe however without the antagonistic impact.

When you have type 2 diabetes, physical action is an essential part of your treatment arrangement. It's likewise essential to have a solid feast arrange and keep up your blood glucose level through solutions or insulin, if important. If that you stay fit and dynamic for the duration of your life, you'll have the capacity to better control your diabetes and keep your blood glucose level in the right range. Controlling your blood glucose level is fundamental to anticipating long haul difficulties, for example, nerve torment and kidney ailment.

Exercise has such a variety of advantages, however the greatest one is that it makes it less demanding to control your blood (glucose) level. Individuals with type 2 diabetes have an excessive amount of glucose in their blood, either because their body doesn't sufficiently deliver insulin to process it, or because their body doesn't utilize insulin legitimately (insulin safe).

In either case, activity can lessen the glucose in your blood. Muscles can utilize glucose without insulin when you're working out. At the end of the day, it doesn't make a difference in case you're insulin safe or if that you don't have enough insulin: when you work out, your muscles get the glucose they require, and thusly, your blood glucose level goes down.

In case you're insulin safe, practice really makes your insulin more compelling. That is—your insulin resistance goes down when you work out, and your cells can utilize the glucose all the more adequately. Activity can likewise individuals with type 2 diabetes maintain a strategic distance from long haul confusions, particularly heart issues. Individuals with diabetes are vulnerable to creating blocked conduits (arteriosclerosis), which can prompt a heart assault. Exercise keeps your heart sound and solid. In addition, exercise offers you some assistance with maintaining great cholesterol—and that offers you some assistance with avoiding arteriosclerosis.

Also, there are all the customary advantages of activity:

Lower pulse

Better control of weight

Greater level of good cholesterol (HDL)

Leaner, more grounded muscles

More grounded bones

More vitality

Enhanced state of mind

Better rest

Stress administration

Be that as it may, Before You Begin Exercising...

At the point when the vast majority are determined to have type 2 diabetes, they are overweight, so the thought of practicing is especially overwhelming. For your wellbeing, you need to begin on a decent, sensible activity arrangement, yet initially, you ought to converse with your specialist.

Your specialist will have the capacity to check your heart wellbeing, which is especially imperative if that you as of now have blocked supply routes or hypertension. You likewise need to mull over whatever other diabetes-related inconveniences—retinopathy or neuropathy, for instance. As you start an activity program, your specialist can allude you to an activity physiologist or diabetes instructor to offer you some assistance with figuring out the best practice program that permits you to get fit as a fiddle for your wellness level.

Additionally before you start working out, you have to set reasonable objectives. If that you haven't practiced much as of late, you will need to begin moderate and step by step build the sum and force of the movement.

Keep in mind to stay hydrated by drinking water and dependably have a treatment for low blood glucose helpful (a 15 g carb nibble is a smart thought). It is keen to check your glucose with your glucose meter previously, then after the fact activity to ensure you are in a sheltered extent.

Being determined to have type 2 diabetes changes your life, however rolling out little improvements to your routine can help you consolidate more physical movement into your day. You have to do what works for your body and your way of life. See the recommendations underneath for what types of activity to do.

Permit yourself some an opportunity to develop to an unfaltering, testing exercise schedule. Furthermore, be alright with going moderate—it's better for your body over the long haul.

What Kinds of Exercise to Do

There are three principle sorts of activity—oxygen consuming, quality preparing, and adaptability work. You ought to plan to have a decent adjust of every one of the three.

Oxygen consuming Exercises

Oxygen consuming activities include:

Strolling

Running/Running

Tennis

Ball

Swimming

Biking

You ought to mean to get no less than 30 minutes of oxygen consuming practice most days of the week. If that you surmise that you can't discover 30 minutes, you can separate the activity into pieces—10 minutes here and there. Develop to 30 minutes bit by bit.

Likewise, extend your innovativeness with regards to fitting in activity. Go out for a stroll at lunch, or get the entire family out after supper for a session of b-ball. Keep in mind that strolling your pooch is a type of activity. Taking the stairs is activity. Strolling from your auto and into the store is activity—so stop more remote away.

You have to figure out how to practice that you really appreciate—because if that it's not fun, you won't do it. It'll harder to stay inspired, regardless of the possibility that you know every one of the advantages of activity. Consider taking gathering classes at the exercise center, or discover a companion to walk or keep running with. Having another person practicing with you makes it more fun and inspiring.

Quality Training

When you have possessed the capacity to incorporate vigorous action into your days, then you can begin including quality preparing.

Quality preparing gives you incline, productive muscles, and it additionally offers you some assistance with maintaining solid, sound bones. It's decent for you when you have type 2 diabetes because muscles utilize the most glucose, so if that you can utilize them all the more, then you'll better ready to control your blood glucose level.

Weight preparing is a standout amongst the most utilized quality preparing systems, despite the fact that you can likewise utilize your own body weight to develop quality—consider force ups and push-ups. When you're beginning a weight preparing program, ensure you know how to utilize all the gear. Ask the staff at your rec center how you ought to appropriately utilize the weights, or think about getting as a fitness coach to take in the best activities for you.

Lifting weights for 20-30 minutes a few times each week is adequate to get the full advantages of quality preparing.

Adaptability Training

With adaptability preparing, you'll enhance how well your muscles and joints work. Extending prior and then afterward work out (particularly after activity) decreases muscle soreness and really unwinds your muscles.

Make a guarantee to work out; make it a need. Your long haul wellbeing relies on upon it, so as intense as it might be to discover time or to rouse yourself to work out, keep at it. It will offer you some assistance with losing weight (if that you have to do that), and it will make your body more productive at utilizing its insulin and glucose.

Exercise is certain to be on your schedule if that you have diabetes. Begin with these go-to tips:

1. Make a rundown of fun exercises. You have bunches of choices, and you don't need to go to an exercise center. What sounds great? Consider something you've for a long while been itching to attempt or something you appreciated previously. Sports, moving, yoga, strolling, and swimming are a couple of thoughts. Anything that raises your heart rate numbers.

2. Get your specialist's OK. Tell them what you need to do. They can ensure you're prepared for it. They'll additionally verify whether you have to change your suppers, insulin, or diabetes pharmaceuticals. Your specialist can likewise fill you in as to whether the season of day you practice matters.

3. Check your glucose. Inquire as to whether you ought to check it before activity. If that you plan to work out for 60 minutes, check your glucose levels frequently during your workout, so you'll know whether you require a nibble. Check your glucose after each workout, with the goal that you can modify if necessary.

The 7-Minute Workout

4. Convey carbs. Continuously keep a little starch nibble, similar to organic product or a natural product drink, available if that your glucose gets low.

5. Guide into it. In case you're not dynamic now, begin with 10 minutes of activity at once. Continuously work up to 30 minutes a day.

6. Quality train at any rate twice every week. It can enhance glucose control. You can lift weights or work with resistance groups. On the other hand you can do moves like push-ups, lurches, and squats, which utilize your own particular body weight.

7. Make it a propensity. Work out, eat, and take your solutions in the meantime every day to avert low glucose, additionally called hypoglycemia.

8. Open up to the world. Work out with somebody who knows you have diabetes and comprehends what to do if your glucose gets too low. It's better time, as well. Additionally wear a restorative distinguishing proof tag, or convey a card that says you have diabetes, to be safe.

9. Regard your feet. Wear athletic shoes that are fit as a fiddle and are the right type for your action. Case in point, don't run in sneakers, because your foot needs an alternate type of backing when you run. Check and clean your feet day by day. Fill your specialist in as to whether you see any new foot issues.

10. Hydrate. Drink water some time recently, during, and after activity.

11. Stop if something all of a sudden damages. If that your muscles are somewhat sore, that is ordinary. Sudden torment isn't. You're not liable to get harmed unless you do excessively, too early.

 Best and Worst Meals for Diabetes-Savvy Dining

10 Health Benefits You'll Get

Keep in mind the amount of activity accomplishes for you, including:

Offers your body some assistance with using insulin, which controls your glucose

Smolders additional muscle to fat ratio ratios

Fortifies muscles and bones

Brings down circulatory strain

Cuts LDL ("awful") cholesterol

Raises HDL ("great") cholesterol

Enhances blood stream

Makes coronary illness and stroke more outlandish

Supports vitality and disposition

Tames stress

How Does Exercise Affect Blood Sugar?

When you work out, your body needs additional vitality from glucose, likewise called glucose.

When you accomplish something rapidly, similar to a sprint to get the transport, your muscles and liver discharge glucose for fuel.

The enormous result comes when you do moderate activity for a more extended time, similar to a climb. Your muscles take up a great deal more glucose when you do that. This brings down your glucose levels.

In case you're doing extreme work out, your glucose levels might rise, incidentally, after you stop.Now and again, it might appear simpler to pop a pill or even take a shot than to put on your strolling shoes and hit the trail. Yet, actually work out, in mix with a solid eating regimen, is one of the best things you can do to deal with yourself if that you have diabetes.

Why exercise?

Exercise smolders calories, which will offer you some assistance with losing weight or keep up a solid weight. Normal activity can offer your body some assistance with responding to insulin and is known not viable in overseeing blood glucose. Activity can bring down blood glucose and potentially lessen the measure of solution you have to treat diabetes, or even dispense with the requirement for pharmaceutical.

Activity can enhance your dissemination, particularly in your arms and legs, where individuals with diabetes can have issues.

Activity can diminish your cholesterol and hypertension. Elevated cholesterol and hypertension can prompt a heart assault or stroke.

Exercise decreases stress, which can raise your glucose level.

It can bring down your danger for coronary illness, decrease your cholesterol levels and your pulse. In a few individuals, exercise joined with a dinner arrangement, can control Type 2 Diabetes without the requirement for drugs.

Step by step instructions to begin working out

In case you're rusty or have as of late been analyzed as having diabetes, see your specialist before you start an activity program. Your specialist can let you know about the sorts of activity that are beneficial for you relying upon how well your diabetes is controlled and any entanglements or different conditions you might have. Here are a few tips for beginning:

In case you're wanting to walk or run, make sure your shoes fit well and are intended for the movement you have personality a top priority. Be ready for rankles. Wear new shoes for somewhat every day until they're agreeable and not as prone to cause rankles. Keep in mind, dependably wear socks.

Begin gradually with a low-effect practice, for example, strolling, swimming, or biking.

Develop the time you spend practicing continuously. If that you need to, begin with five minutes and include a touch of time every day.

Continuously wear an ID tag demonstrating that you have diabetes to protect legitimate treatment if that there's an issue when you're practicing or you have a harm. Abstain from lifting overwhelming weights as a precautionary measure against sudden hypertension.

If that you have foot issues, consider swimming or biking, which is less demading on the feet than running. Stretch for five minutes previously, then after the fact your workout paying little respect to how extreme you plan to work out.

How frequently would it be a good idea for you to work out?

Attempt to practice in the meantime consistently for the same term. This will control your glucose. Exercise no less than three times each week for around 30 to 45 minutes.

Shouldn't something be said about nourishment and insulin?

If that you plan to practice over an hour in the wake of eating, it's a smart thought to have a nibble. By and large, it's great to have a high-starch nibble, for example, six ounces of natural product juice or half of a plain bbagel.

In case you're doing substantial practice, for example, vigorous exercise, running or handball, you might need to eat more, for example, a half of a meat sandwich and some milk.

If that you haven't eaten for 60 minutes or if your glucose is under 100 to 120, eat or drink something like an apple or a glass of milk before you work out. Convey a nibble with you if there should be an occurrence of low glucose.

If that you utilize insulin, exercise subsequent to eating, not some time recently. Test your glucose some time recently, during and subsequent to working out. Try not to practice when your glucose is more than 240.

In case you're not an insulin client, test your glucose prior and then afterward practicing if that you take pills for diabetes.

At the point when is activity an issue?

If that your glucose level is more than 300 mg/dl, if that you are wiped out, shy of breath, have ketones in your pee or are encountering any shivering, agony or deadness in your legs, don't work out. Additionally if your pharmaceutical is cresting, it's better not to work out.

Insulin response and exercise

Treat it when you feel it. Try not to hold up. Make sure you have a few raisins or treat close by to raise your blood glucose level.

Activities to Avoid When You Have Diabetes

Consistent physical action is an imperative part of a sound way of life when you have diabetes. It is useful for your cardiovascular framework and can control blood glucose levels. Be that as it may, there are times when you should be watchful about practicing with diabetes. If that you have certain diabetes confusions, there are activities that you ought to maintain a strategic distance from. Michael See, MS, RCEP, Clinical Exercise Physiologist at Joslin Diabetes Center, talks about specific circumstances that might oblige you to adjust your work out regime

The accompanying confusions might influence your activity schedule:.

Proliferative diabetic retinopathy (PDR)— Patients with diabetes and dynamic PDR ought to stay away from exercises that include strenuous lifting; unforgiving, high-effect exercises; or putting the head in a transformed position for amplified timeframes.

Diabetic fringe neuropathy—Diabetic fringe neuropathy might bring about loss of sensation and position attention to your feet. Tedious activity on uncaring feet can prompt ulceration and breaks. "Limit your decision of activity to low effect or non-weight bearing exercises," says See.

Propelled kidney sickness—Individuals with diabetes and propelled kidney illness can participate in moderate force exercises, however ought to maintain a strategic distance from strenuous movement.

High blood glucose levels—Individuals with type 1 diabetes ought to dodge exercise if fasting blood glucose is higher than 250 mg/dl and ketones are available. Alert ought to be utilized if glucose levels are higher than 300 and no ketones are available. People with type 2 diabetes ought to maintain a strategic distance from activity if blood glucose is higher than 400 mg/dl. Observing blood glucose some time recently, after and perhaps during physical movement is important to keep blood glucose inside of a fitting extent.

Continuously counsel with an activity or medicinal services proficient before starting any work out program.

Chapter 8

Step by step instructions to cure diabetes

Have you or a relative simply gotten a prediabetes finding? This is a genuine reminder, yet it doesn't need to mean diabetes will create. You can find a way to turn things around.

It's a chance to begin lifestyle changes or medicines, and moderate or even avoid diabetes, says Gregg Gerety, MD, head of endocrinology at St. Diminish's Hospital in Albany, NY. These progressions to natural, day by day propensities are a decent approach to begin.

Move more. Hands down, activity is one of the best things you can do to make diabetes more outlandish. "Physical movement is a crucial part of the treatment arrangement for prediabetes in light of the fact that it brings down blood glucose levels and diminishes muscle to fat ratio ratios," says Patti B. Geil, an enlisted dietitian and co-creator of What Do I Eat Now? A Step-by-Step Guide to Eating Right With Type 2 Diabetes.

If you haven't practiced in a while, begin by building more action into your day. Step set up during TV ads. In a perfect world, you ought to practice no less than 30 minutes a day, 5 days a week. Tell your specialist about your activity arranges. what's more, inquire as to whether you ought to consider any unique variables or constraints.

Great to Know

How would you keep your glucose enduring for the duration of the day?

I observe that avoiding carbs for breakfast sets the tone for my suppers during the rest .

Get in shape.
If you're overweight, you won't not need to lose as much as you think to have any kind of effect. In one late study, individuals who had prediabetes and lost 5% to 7% of their body weight (only 10 to 14 pounds for somebody who weighs 200 pounds) trimmed their odds of creating diabetes more than half.

Check in all the more frequently.
A decent general guideline is to see your specialist each 3 to 6 months, Gerety says. The result is twofold: If you're doing great, you get encouraging feedback from your specialist. Furthermore, if the condition is not going so well, your specialist can offer you some assistance with getting on track.

Venture up to better nourishment.
Geil recommends a few ways you can enhance your eating routine. Load up on vegetables, particularly the less boring sorts, for example, spinach, broccoli, carrots, and green beans. Go for no less than three servings a day. Add all the more high-fiber sustenances to your suppers. Appreciate organic product with some restraint, around one to three servings for each day. What's more, pick entire grains over handled grains. For instance, eat cocoa rice rather than white rice.

Additionally, swap fatty nourishments. "Drink skim drain instead of entire milk, diet pop as opposed to standard pop," Geil says. "Pick lower-fat variants of cheddar, yogurt, and plate of mixed greens dressings."

Infrequent snacks are fine as well, however exchange the high-fat, fatty chips and sweets for new organic product, or entire wheat saltines with nutty spread or low-fat cheddar, Geil says.

Make rest a need. A lot of value close eye is key for some reasons, however not getting enough think about a customary premise plays destruction with your wellbeing - and your weight. Too little rest makes shedding pounds harder, says Theresa Garnero, a diabetes medical caretaker instructor and creator of Your First Year With Diabetes: What to Do, Month by Month. A rest deficiency additionally makes it harder for your body to utilize insulin viably and might make diabetes more probable.

Make some great rest propensities and stay with them. Go to quaint little inn up in the meantime consistently. Unwind before you turn out the lights. Try not to stare at the TV or utilize your tech gadgets when you're attempting to nod off.

The right personality set and backing can offer you some assistance with making a change. Here's the manner by which to begin.

Pick and submit.
Acknowledge that you won't do things flawlessly consistently, yet vow to do your best more often than not. "Settle on a cognizant decision to be steady with regular exercises that are to the greatest advantage of your wellbeing," Garnero says. "Let yourself know, 'I'm going to put

forth a valiant effort. I'm going to roll out little improvements after some time.'"

Get support.

Getting more fit, eating sound dinners, and practicing frequently are less demanding if you have individuals who consider you responsible, says Ronald T. Ackermann, MD, MPH. Join a gathering to be in the organization of others with comparable objectives.

Eat Fat - A Step-by-Step Guide to Low Carb Living

"Is a low fat eating routine bravo?" Most of us will without a doubt say yes, yet is this truly the case? It is all around reported that the issue of stoutness is developing over the world, with it comes the greater danger of:

Coronary illness, strokes and greasy liver

Diabetes (Type 2) — which has quickly turned into a worldwide plague

A few diseases (endometrial, bosom, and colon)

There is developing proof which demonstrates that the well known low fat/high sugar eating routine is really a myth and that it might be fuelling the heftiness and Type 2 diabetes pestilences. Our scientist have identified that a low carb, high fat lifestyle can pulsate executioner conditions like diabetes, coronary illness, epilepsy, tumor and dementia and even back off the maturing process.

UK-prestigious pro, Dr Trudi Deakin (our Chief Executive) says that this six-stage arrangement will give new would like to individuals who are overweight or are experiencing a long haul wellbeing condition. A low carb/high fat lifestyle can individuals to get more fit and control heftiness, diabetes, coronary illness and numerous other wellbeing conditions.

We have likewise identified that eating sugar increments blood glucose levels, which then builds the levels of a hormone called insulin in the blood. This hormone advances weight pick up, forestalls weight reduction and adds to other wellbeing issues. Eating abundance carbs additionally builds the awful levels of cholesterol particles in the blood. Conditions, for example, corpulence, Type 2 diabetes and coronary illness can be counteracted if the arrangement is received. Indeed, even the individuals who as of now have the conditions might find that their condition is switched with the right lifestyle.

Q) I have a festival this weekend so there will be some liquor included. Inquiry is, what is best to drink instead of lager?
A) Spirits with without sugar blenders (thin line tonic, diet coke or abstain from food lemonade) or dry white wine or red wine. Page 51 in the low carb handbook gives the carb substance of a few liquor drinks that might offer assistance.

Q) Can you suggest any sauces? Is there any sort of low carb tomato sauce, or perhaps a cheddar sauce to put over my cauliflower?
A) Trudi: If I make a tomato-based sauce, I add passata to fricasseed onions, peppers, mushrooms and so on. If I make cheddar sauce, I either soften full fat cream cheddar in a pot and include ground cheddar (in addition to a touch of water if too thick) or melt spread in a pan, add somewhat stock before including twofold cream and cheddar.

Q) Regarding passata, do you mean puree as opposed to genuine tomatoes, as resembles the tomatoes contain a great deal of carbs/sugar?

A) Yes tomatoes do contain a few carbs however passata more often than not has significantly less carbs (and added substances) than tomato based sauces such Ragu and Dolmio. This one (see join) has 4.3g carbs per 100g – if the jug served 4 individuals, you would get 5.4g carbs, which is effectively consolidated into a low carb diet.

Q) There are heaps of low carb administrations out there, and they all appear to be marginally different. E.g. Yours says peas are OK; others say no in light of the fact that they're excessively carby/sweet; yours says little measures of red wine is OK, others say wine is a flat out no-no due to the sugar content. Yours says eating routine coke's OK; others say no chance. So I'm somewhat befuddled about which "runs" I ought to be taking after?
An) All our data is exceptional and proof based to the best of our insight at the season of print. We utilize the Carbs and Cals books for sugar content which advises that a 80g bit of peas contain 8g of carbs and hence this can be incorporated into the 50g every day recompense if fancied. The red wine data demonstrates that it contains next to no starch (~1g per 125ml glass) despite the fact that be cautious with lower liquor or sweet wines as these will contain more carbs.

We understanding that clashing messages might be mistaking for you. We would love reliable data to be given to people in general. It might be because of the way that individuals without the important dietary ability are giving guidance yet tragically there is nothing we can do about this.

Q) Is it alright to prepare with soya protein separately?
A) Be mindful so as not to exaggerate Soya Protein Isolate. It is 90-95% protein and 100g of protein can be changed over to 56g glucose so eating protein to abundance can even now spike your glucose and insulin levels.

Q) How would you cook with coconut flour?
A) You require far less coconut flour than grain-based flour, so for each one measure of grain-based flour in a formula utilize only one-quarter to 33% measure of coconut flour. You ought to additionally add in one egg for every ounce of coconut flour to assume the position of gluten and tie the blend together. If you don't have eggs close by, you can likewise include hemp powder, chia seeds or ground flax seeds (one tablespoon in three tablespoons of water makes a substitute for one egg) to tie the coconut flour together.

If you're utilizing coconut flour as a part of a common grain-based flour formula, you'll have to analyze a bit to get the extents simply right. Including pretty much coconut flour will offer you some assistance with getting the composition you cherish, and including the right blend of tying fixings, (for example, eggs or flax seed) will guarantee the prepared great doesn't just go into disrepair. Coconut flour really works extraordinary as a thickening operators in formulas too, because of its high sponginess. Have a go at adding coconut flour to soups, stews, or smoothies for a rich, generous composition.

Q) I am pondering what the impacts of a low carb/high fat eating regimen would be on entrail wellbeing particularly somebody who is clogged up and on danger of gut malignancy additionally on those with lower body weight?

A) Constipation –

at first patients might report stoppage as this is as often as possible an issue when individuals change their eating regimen. On the other hand, this soon determines as the fiber consumption doesn't need to be lower if individuals get the right instruction and devour adequate liquids, veg, berries, nuts, flaxseed, coconut flour and so forth. Dietary fat can likewise act as a purgative.

Inside malignancy –

there is rising examination taking a gander at LCHF diets for backing off the development of disease as hyperinsulinemia and glucose can empower development of tumor cells. Epidemiological studies have presumed that red meat might bring about inside tumor yet there are numerous constraints particularly as observational studies can't identify circumstances and end results furthermore they have not isolated plant cultivated cows from grass-bolstered dairy cattle raised without hormones and anti-infection agents. Additionally diminishing omega-6 unsaturated fats (prepared vegetable oils) might likewise lessen disease hazard.

Lower body weight –

the high fat nature of the eating regimen permits individuals to expend a more vitality thick eating routine without feeling bloated. Notwithstanding, I have not go over anybody that wishes to increment weight. It typically works by making individuals feel more full for more and in this manner making them more averse to nibble between suppers which might vanquish the article if somebody is attempting to put on weight.

Q) Would it be proper for somebody who is very overweight however does long separation swimming?

A) The LCHF eating routine is awesome for anybody doing continuance sports. It takes 3-6 weeks to change over i.e. adjust to using fat rather than carbs, however once they improve continuance (even an incline individual can have 135,000 calories of put away fat though they can just have around 2,000 calories of put away carbs) and weight reduction.

Q) I have been determined to have crainiopharaginoma which has abandoned me with complex hormone issues and I've been told I will discover it extremely difficult to get more fit. I've attempted various of eating regimens and I can't discover any that appear to work!

A) Trudi: I don't know all that much about crainiopharaginoma yet from what I've quite recently perused on patient.co.uk, I comprehend that weight is high at around half of patients. I am expecting that the thyroxine is effectively treating the hypothyroidism? Additionally, do you need to be on steroids (hydrocortisone)? Steroids advance weight pick up. It might be worth inquiring as to whether there is another drug you can take.

Surely the low carb high fat dietary methodology might offer assistance. As dinners with for all intents and purposes no carbs and elevated amounts of fat are additionally fulfilling and filling, a great many people find that they can dispose of all snacks and can regularly oversee on 2 suppers for each day. This dietary methodology decreases blood levels of the hormone insulin. Insulin is the thing that we call a weight advancing hormone – it urges us to store fat and forestalls us smoldering it for vitality. Insulin levels raise when we eat sugar and along these lines if we overlook carbs, levels of insulin drop and empower weight reduction.

Q) One issue which I have dependably had when I have attempted low carb is sufficient fiber
A) When individuals at first embrace a LCHF diet they might encounter stoppage however the body soon adjusts. Dietary fat really stools movement. Meanwhile – ensure you are sufficiently dynamic, keep on drinking a lot of liquid and ensure that you have adequate green verdant vegetables.

Q) Are there any arrangements to discharge the above book in e-position (ignite/pdf or whatever) by any stretch of the imagination?
A) We are at present investigating discharging the "Eat Fat: Step-by-Step Guide to Low Carb Living" as a digital book. It would be ideal if you be patient and we'll dispatch when we can.

Q) Will receiving a low carb high fat (LCHF) lifestyle help my polycystic ovaries?
A) People with polycystic ovary disorder frequently have insulin resistance and this outcomes in abnormal amounts of insulin in the blood. Insulin is a weight advancing hormone that empowers fat capacity - it sends signs to the fat cells, instructing them to store fat and to clutch the fat that they as of now convey. Along these lines individuals with abnormal amounts of insulin frequently battle to keep

up or get more fit. An greater waist boundary is one which is troublesome.

www.ingramcontent.com/pod-product-compliance
Lightning Source LLC
Chambersburg PA
CBHW020414290526
45785CB00002B/550